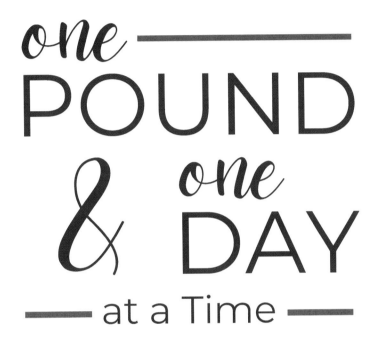

one
POUND
& one
DAY
—— at a Time ——

Weight Loss Journey

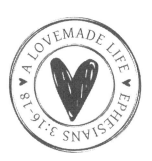

A Lovemade Life was created to encourage women to live by faith, live in love, and to love life. If you would like to be encouraged in faith, relationships, and personal growth, you can connect with A Lovemade Life on Facebook and Instagram.

This book has been created with time, attention to detail, effort, and love.

Occasionally, mistakes can happen in printing. If you have any issues with the quality of this book- binding, printing errors, etc., please contact me at: jenstadler@alovemadelife.com

You can return the faulty one (free of charge) for a replacement.

For questions, suggestions, or feedback related to this product, please feel free to contact me at: jenstadler@alovemadelife.com.

If you find value in this product, please consider sharing that value with others by leaving a review on Amazon.

SEE OTHER BOOKS OFFERED
FROM OUR PUBLISHING PLATFORMS

Visit A Lovemade Life's Author Central Page

Visit Box Book Publishing's Author Central Page

CONGRATULATIONS! You've just taken the first step toward a healthier you. You made a decision and you took action. That's what it takes to accomplish any goal.

Maybe this is your first weight-loss attempt, or like many women, you've lost count of the number of times you've tried. Do you know the most important part? You're still trying! Failure is for those who quit trying. You bought this book, which means you just showed up. You're here and you're ready!

Don't wait until you've reached your goal to be proud of yourself.
Be proud of every step you take toward reaching your goal.

Obviously, you're not where you want to be with your weight or your body (because you bought this book). But, you're on your way and this book will help you get there. It includes all the tools you need to evaluate, plan, and track your progress toward a healthier you! Be consistent with answering the journal prompts and with tracking your daily information. Doing so will help you stay focused and motivated. The easier you can implement something into your day to day, the more likely you are to stick with it in the long run.

Maybe you don't have time to spend hours at the gym or working out at home. Just find ways to move your body and be active that work for you- walking in the neighborhood, dancing, or playing with your kids. The important thing is to keep your body as active as possible. If you love a traditional workout, great. On the other hand, if you view it as an impossibility to fit into your day or as a torturous affair, you're only going to feel miserable and lose motivation. Find something active that you love to do and do it. Any movement/activity is good for your body. You may also discover as you get healthier, your body will **want** to do more.

While activity is crucial to your overall health and fitness, the majority of weight loss happens in the kitchen. *If you eat what you've always eaten, you will weigh what you've always weighed.*

Few people succeed long-term with sudden and drastic changes to their diets. Focus on small changes. Choose foods that work for you, not against you. Once you've changed one habit, create another one. You don't have to be extreme, just consistent. Focus not just on losing weight, but on establishing a new, healthier lifestyle.

This book was created not just to give you practical tools to help you create a healthier you, but to inspire and motivate you along the way. There are weekly and monthly trackers in the back of the book. Choose the ones that work best for you. I hope you fall in love with taking care of your body. Remember- sustainable, long-term weight-loss is a marathon, not a sprint.

It took more than a day to put the weight on. It will take more than a day to take it off.
But, you can do it - one day and one pound at a time!

Tips & Strategies

PRACTICALITY

· Find what works for you - everyone's circumstances are different.
· Practice portion control.
· Use smaller plates.
· Chew slowly.
· Drink water, especially before each meal.
· Stop mindless eating (in front of the TV or computer) - pay attention to what you're eating.
· Set a deadline (at night) to stop eating (e.g. don't eat after 7pm).
· Eat the healthy foods on your plate first.
· Get support from a close friend or a family member.
· Plan ahead with meals and snacks (prep and you'll be prepared).
· Reduce stress to eliminate emotional eating.
· Get adequate sleep.

POSITIVITY

· Focus on what you "will do," not on what you won't do.
   (Focus first on increasing good foods and less on decreasing bad foods.)
· Maintain a positive mindset. Your body hears everything your mind says.
· Post positive and motivating messages where you will see them regularly.
· Don't dwell on negative thoughts. Give them a moment and let them go.
· Practice forgiving yourself. Mistakes and setbacks will happen - refocus.
· Remember your goals and why you set them.
· Don't let the scale undermine your motivation. Weight fluctuates - there are other measures of success: the way you feel, energy, sleep, the fit of clothes, healthier skin and a clear complexion, etc.
· Read books, blogs, magazines, etc. that promote a healthy lifestyle. Surround yourself with inspiration and motivation.

PROGRESS

· Be specific with your goals. Vague goals are difficult to achieve.
· Set short-term AND long-term goals. Create non-food rewards.
· Set realistic and achievable goals so you see progress.
· Create a sensible timeline for achieving your goals. Consider how your day to day life will affect your timeline.
· "It's a slow process, but quitting won't speed it up." - unknown

*These tips and strategies are from personal experience only and are not to be taken as professional or medical advice.

the Old Me

Add a current photo of yourself.

What are some things you really love about yourself?

Stop hating yourself for everything you aren't.
Start loving yourself for everything you are.

Old & New Habits

What is a habit? What are your habits? How do your behaviors affect your habits?

Miriam-Webster defines a habit as *a usual way of behaving : something that a person does often in a regular and repeated way.*

Habits are established from our repeated behaviors. Unfortunately, many of us gain weight or fail to care for our bodies because we engage in repeated behaviors that establish bad habits. Many people start their weight-loss journey just trying to stop bad behaviors/habits. The key to successful weight-loss and long-term lifestyle change is to **replace** your old habits with new ones.

How will you do that?
1. Evaluate your current bad habits.
2. Determine new habits to replace the old ones. (See strategies below.)
3. Consistently track your habits and progress.

TIPS & STRATEGIES

· Identify triggers for your bad habits.
· Remove temptations from your environment. Keep healthy snacks accessible.
· Focus on building one new habit at a time. Be specific about the habit.
   (Instead of "I'll eat more vegetables," make it "I'll eat two vegetables at meal time.")
· Start with easy habits you can establish without a lot of motivation.
   Set yourself up for success.
· Break habits down into smaller sections. It's easier to start doing 10 pushups 2x/day
   than to do 20 pushups at one time. Make it manageable.
· Make small increases to your new habits. Small changes add up over time. Don't
   overwhelm yourself and undermine your motivation.
· Focus on consistency, not perfection. Expect to struggle, but keep going. Habits are
   formed by consistent behavior.
· Habits are more easily formed when they can be triggered by routine (e.g. taking your
   vitamins with breakfast, taking a walk right after dinner, etc.)

Good or bad, habits always deliver results.
- Jack Canfield

My Habits

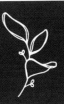

What are 3-4 old habits I would like to change?

_____
_____
_____
_____

How are these habits harming my health or well-being?

_____
_____
_____
_____

What new habits would I like to establish?

_____
_____
_____
_____

In what ways will these new habits benefit my health and well-being?

_____
_____
_____
_____

Your habits will determine your future.
- Jack Canfield

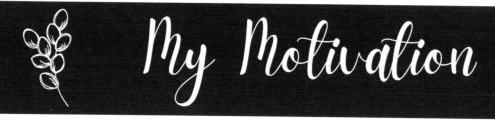

My Motivation

How will taking care of myself enable me to take better care of others?

_____

_____

_____

_____

_____

What are some ways losing weight and being healthier will improve my life?

_____

_____

_____

_____

_____

*What is my ultimate motivation for losing weight and being healthier?

_____

_____

_____

_____

_____

* Something to consider: Losing weight and "looking better" may be a desire, but those results take time to achieve.
Many people struggle to maintain motivation in the short-term, while waiting for those results.
People sometimes find it easier to maintain motivation by focusing on more immediate motivators-
having more energy, sleeping better, feeling better, etc.

Goals & Rewards

GOAL 1

_____

Accomplished ☐

My Reward

_____

Steps to take

_____
_____
_____
_____

GOAL 2

_____

Accomplished ☐

My Reward

_____

Steps to take

_____
_____
_____
_____

GOAL 3

_____

Accomplished ☐

My Reward

_____

Steps to take

_____
_____
_____
_____

GOAL 4

_____

Accomplished ☐

My Reward

_____

Steps to take

_____
_____
_____
_____

Every accomplishment begins with the decision to try.

Goals & Rewards

GOAL 5

Steps to take

_____

Accomplished ☐

My Reward

_____

GOAL 6

Steps to take

_____

Accomplished ☐

My Reward

_____

GOAL 7

Steps to take

_____

Accomplished ☐

My Reward

_____

GOAL 8

Steps to take

_____

Accomplished ☐

My Reward

_____

If the plan doesn't work, change the plan not the goal.

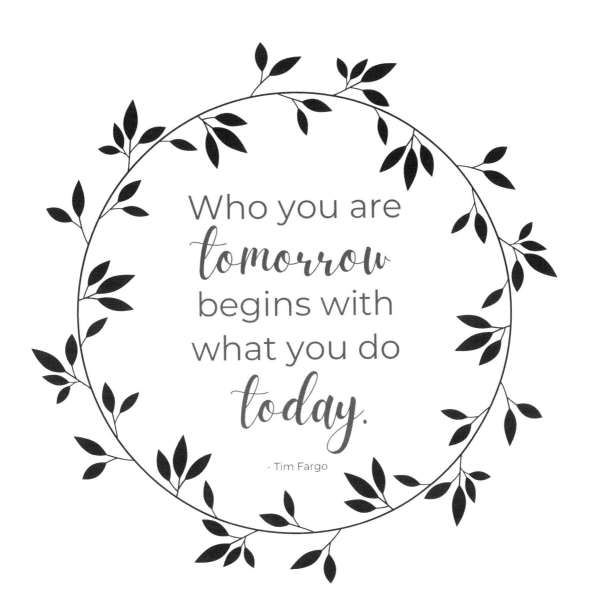

Who you are *tomorrow* begins with what you do *today*.

- Tim Fargo

MY GOAL FOR THIS WEEK

_____

STEPS I WILL TAKE

_____

_____

_____

Week One

Body Measurements

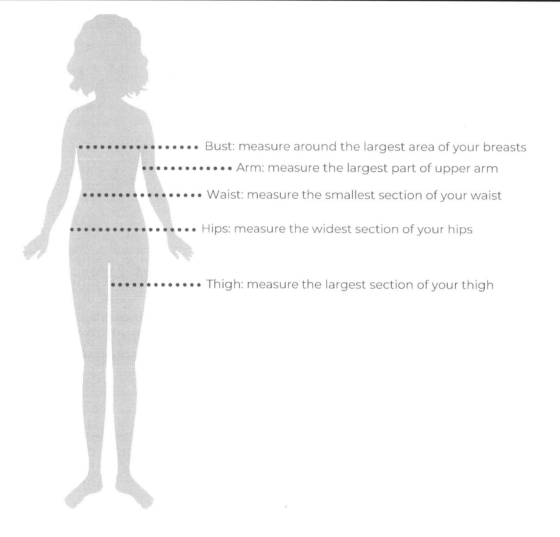

Bust: measure around the largest area of your breasts

Arm: measure the largest part of upper arm

Waist: measure the smallest section of your waist

Hips: measure the widest section of your hips

Thigh: measure the largest section of your thigh

TIPS FOR TAKING BODY MEASUREMENTS

· Wear tight fitting clothes or no clothes when you take measurements.
· Try to measure at the same areas each time (e.g. near the same freckle, etc.).
· Use a good quality measuring tape.
· Record your measurements so you can track your changes over time.

Beauty comes from the heart, not the mirror.
- Unknown

Week 1 - A New Beginning

Date

Starting Weight

My Goal Weight

Starting Measurements

Bust

Waist

Arm

Thigh

Hips

Reasons
I want to lose weight...

the difference between your body this week and your body next week is what you do for the next seven days to achieve your goals.
- Unknown

	Breakfast	Lunch	Dinner	Snacks
Monday				
Tuesday				
Wednesday				
Thursday				
Friday				
Saturday				
Sunday				

Week One / Meal Plan

Date _____ Monday

Sleep

7pm · 8 · 9 · 10 · 11 · 12am · 1 · 2 · 3 · 4 · 5 · 6 · 7 · 8 · 9 · 10 · 11 · 12pm

Quality: ☆☆☆☆☆   Hours: _____   Energy Level: ☆☆☆☆☆

Mood

cheerful   sad   excited   worried   stressed
upset   angry   frustrated   content   indifferent

Meals

BREAKFAST

LUNCH

DINNER

SNACKS

Misc.

WATER: ⬜⬜⬜⬜⬜⬜⬜⬜

VITAMINS / SUPPLEMENTS ☐

STEPS: _____

OTHER: _____

Exercise

ACTIVITY	DISTANCE / REPS / TIME

Cardio ☐   Strength ☐
Stretching ☐   Other ☐

Notes

Date _____

Sleep

7pm · 8 · 9 · 10 · 11 · 12am · 1 · 2 · 3 · 4 · 5 · 6 · 7 · 8 · 9 · 10 · 11 · 12pm

Quality: ☆☆☆☆☆   Hours: _____   Energy Level: ☆☆☆☆☆

Mood

| cheerful | sad | excited | worried | stressed |
| upset | angry | frustrated | content | indifferent |

Meals

BREAKFAST
_____
_____
_____

LUNCH
_____
_____
_____

DINNER
_____
_____
_____

SNACKS
_____
_____

Misc.

WATER: ▯ ▯ ▯ ▯ ▯ ▯ ▯ ▯

VITAMINS / SUPPLEMENTS ☐

STEPS: _____

OTHER: _____

Exercise

ACTIVITY	DISTANCE / REPS / TIME
_____	_____
_____	_____
_____	_____

Cardio ☐   Strength ☐
Stretching ☐   Other ☐

Notes

_____
_____
_____

Date

_____

Wednesday

Sleep

7pm · 8 · 9 · 10 · 11 · 12am · 1 · 2 · 3 · 4 · 5 · 6 · 7 · 8 · 9 · 10 · 11 · 12pm

Quality: ☆☆☆☆☆   Hours: _____   Energy Level: ☆☆☆☆☆

Mood

| cheerful | sad | excited | worried | stressed |
| upset | angry | frustrated | content | indifferent |

Meals

BREAKFAST
_____
_____
_____
_____

LUNCH
_____
_____
_____

DINNER
_____
_____
_____

SNACKS
_____
_____

Misc.

WATER: ☐ ☐ ☐ ☐ ☐ ☐ ☐ ☐

VITAMINS / SUPPLEMENTS ☐

STEPS: _____

OTHER: _____

Exercise

ACTIVITY	DISTANCE / REPS / TIME
_____	_____
_____	_____
_____	_____
_____	_____

Cardio ☐   Strength ☐

Stretching ☐   Other ☐

Notes

_____
_____
_____
_____

Date

Thursday

Sleep

7pm · 8 · 9 · 10 · 11 · 12am · 1 · 2 · 3 · 4 · 5 · 6 · 7 · 8 · 9 · 10 · 11 · 12pm

Quality: ☆☆☆☆☆   Hours: _____   Energy Level: ☆☆☆☆☆

Mood

| cheerful | sad | excited | worried | stressed |
| upset | angry | frustrated | content | indifferent |

Meals

BREAKFAST
_____
_____
_____

LUNCH
_____
_____
_____

DINNER
_____
_____
_____

SNACKS
_____
_____

Misc.

WATER: ⬜⬜⬜⬜⬜⬜⬜⬜

VITAMINS / SUPPLEMENTS ☐

STEPS: _____

OTHER: _____

Exercise

ACTIVITY	DISTANCE / REPS / TIME
_____	_____
_____	_____
_____	_____

Cardio ☐   Strength ☐
Stretching ☐   Other ☐

Notes

_____
_____
_____

Sleep

7pm · 8 · 9 · 10 · 11 · 12am · 1 · 2 · 3 · 4 · 5 · 6 · 7 · 8 · 9 · 10 · 11 · 12pm

Quality: ☆☆☆☆☆   Hours: _____   Energy Level: ☆☆☆☆☆

Mood

cheerful   sad   excited   worried   stressed
upset   angry   frustrated   content   indifferent

Meals

BREAKFAST
_____
_____
_____
_____

LUNCH
_____
_____
_____

DINNER
_____
_____
_____

SNACKS
_____
_____

Misc.

WATER: ⬜⬜⬜⬜⬜⬜⬜⬜

VITAMINS / SUPPLEMENTS ☐

STEPS: _____

OTHER: _____

Exercise

ACTIVITY	DISTANCE / REPS / TIME
_____	_____
_____	_____
_____	_____

Cardio ☐   Strength ☐
Stretching ☐   Other ☐

Notes

_____
_____
_____
_____

Date

Saturday

Sleep

7pm · 8 · 9 · 10 · 11 · 12am · 1 · 2 · 3 · 4 · 5 · 6 · 7 · 8 · 9 · 10 · 11 · 12pm

Quality: ☆ ☆ ☆ ☆ ☆   Hours: _____   Energy Level: ☆ ☆ ☆ ☆ ☆

Mood

| cheerful | sad | excited | worried | stressed |
| upset | angry | frustrated | content | indifferent |

Meals

BREAKFAST

LUNCH

DINNER

SNACKS

Misc.

WATER: ⬜ ⬜ ⬜ ⬜ ⬜ ⬜ ⬜ ⬜

VITAMINS / SUPPLEMENTS ⬜

STEPS: _____

OTHER: _____

Exercise

ACTIVITY	DISTANCE / REPS / TIME

Cardio ⬜   Strength ⬜

Stretching ⬜   Other ⬜

Notes

Sleep

7pm · 8 · 9 · 10 · 11 · 12am · 1 · 2 · 3 · 4 · 5 · 6 · 7 · 8 · 9 · 10 · 11 · 12pm

Quality: ☆☆☆☆☆   Hours: _____   Energy Level: ☆☆☆☆☆

Mood

| cheerful | sad | excited | worried | stressed |
| upset | angry | frustrated | content | indifferent |

Meals

BREAKFAST

LUNCH

DINNER

SNACKS

Misc.

WATER: 🥛🥛🥛🥛🥛🥛🥛🥛

VITAMINS / SUPPLEMENTS ☐

STEPS: _____

OTHER: _____

Exercise

ACTIVITY	DISTANCE / REPS / TIME

Cardio ☐   Strength ☐
Stretching ☐   Other ☐

Notes

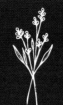 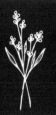

Week 1 Results

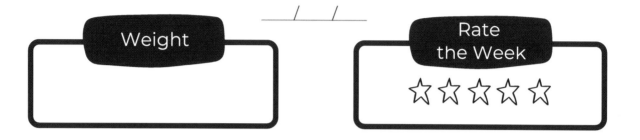

/ /

Weight

Rate the Week

☆ ☆ ☆ ☆ ☆

Write a brief note to yourself, providing encouragement
for the journey ahead.

_____
_____
_____
_____

What worked well this past week?

_____
_____
_____

What was challenging this past week?

_____
_____
_____

What is one thing you can improve this next week?

_____
_____
_____

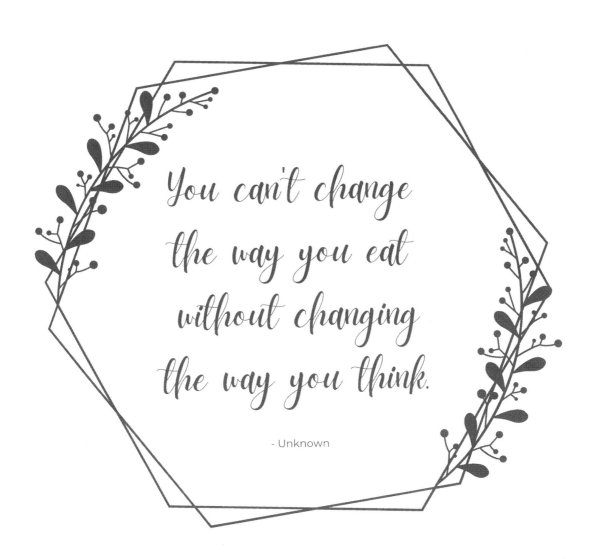

You can't change
the way you eat
without changing
the way you think.

- Unknown

MY GOAL FOR THIS WEEK

_____

STEPS I WILL TAKE

_____

_____

_____

Week Two

	Breakfast	Lunch	Dinner	Snacks
Monday				
Tuesday				
Wednesday				
Thursday				
Friday				
Saturday				
Sunday				

Week Two / Meal Plan

Date

Monday

_____

Sleep

7pm · 8 · 9 · 10 · 11 · 12am · 1 · 2 · 3 · 4 · 5 · 6 · 7 · 8 · 9 · 10 · 11 · 12pm

Quality: ☆☆☆☆☆   Hours: _____   Energy Level: ☆☆☆☆☆

Mood

cheerful   sad   excited   worried   stressed
upset   angry   frustrated   content   indifferent

Meals

BREAKFAST

LUNCH

DINNER

SNACKS

Misc.

WATER: ⬜⬜⬜⬜⬜⬜⬜⬜

VITAMINS / SUPPLEMENTS ☐

STEPS: _____

OTHER: _____

Exercise

ACTIVITY	DISTANCE / REPS / TIME

Cardio ☐   Strength ☐
Stretching ☐   Other ☐

Notes

Date _____ Tuesday

Sleep

7pm · 8 · 9 · 10 · 11 · 12am · 1 · 2 · 3 · 4 · 5 · 6 · 7 · 8 · 9 · 10 · 11 · 12pm

Quality: ☆☆☆☆☆   Hours: _____   Energy Level: ☆☆☆☆☆

Mood

| cheerful | sad | excited | worried | stressed |
| upset | angry | frustrated | content | indifferent |

Meals

BREAKFAST

LUNCH

DINNER

SNACKS

Misc.

WATER: ☐☐☐☐☐☐☐☐

VITAMINS / SUPPLEMENTS ☐

STEPS: _____

OTHER: _____

Exercise

ACTIVITY	DISTANCE / REPS / TIME

Cardio ☐   Strength ☐
Stretching ☐   Other ☐

Notes

Date ❧ ❧ ❧ Wednesday

_____

Sleep

7pm · 8 · 9 · 10 · 11 · 12am · 1 · 2 · 3 · 4 · 5 · 6 · 7 · 8 · 9 · 10 · 11 · 12pm

Quality: ☆ ☆ ☆ ☆ ☆   Hours: _____   Energy Level: ☆ ☆ ☆ ☆ ☆

Mood

cheerful	sad	excited	worried	stressed
upset	angry	frustrated	content	indifferent

Meals

BREAKFAST

LUNCH

DINNER

SNACKS

Misc.

WATER: ⬜ ⬜ ⬜ ⬜ ⬜ ⬜ ⬜ ⬜

VITAMINS / SUPPLEMENTS ☐

STEPS: _____

OTHER: _____

Exercise

ACTIVITY	DISTANCE / REPS / TIME

Cardio ☐   Strength ☐

Stretching ☐   Other ☐

Notes

_____

Sleep

7pm · 8 · 9 · 10 · 11 · 12am · 1 · 2 · 3 · 4 · 5 · 6 · 7 · 8 · 9 · 10 · 11 · 12pm

Quality: ☆☆☆☆☆   Hours: _____   Energy Level: ☆☆☆☆☆

Mood

| cheerful | sad | excited | worried | stressed |
| upset | angry | frustrated | content | indifferent |

Meals

BREAKFAST
_____
_____
_____

LUNCH
_____
_____
_____

DINNER
_____
_____
_____

SNACKS
_____
_____

Misc.

WATER: ▯ ▯ ▯ ▯ ▯ ▯ ▯ ▯

VITAMINS / SUPPLEMENTS ☐

STEPS: _____

OTHER: _____

Exercise

ACTIVITY	DISTANCE / REPS / TIME
_____	_____
_____	_____
_____	_____

Cardio ☐   Strength ☐

Stretching ☐   Other ☐

Notes

_____
_____
_____
_____

Date

_____

Friday

Sleep

7pm · 8 · 9 · 10 · 11 · 12am · 1 · 2 · 3 · 4 · 5 · 6 · 7 · 8 · 9 · 10 · 11 · 12pm

Quality: ☆☆☆☆☆   Hours: _____   Energy Level: ☆☆☆☆☆

Mood

cheerful   sad   excited   worried   stressed

upset   angry   frustrated   content   indifferent

Meals

BREAKFAST

LUNCH

DINNER

SNACKS

Misc.

WATER: ☐ ☐ ☐ ☐ ☐ ☐ ☐ ☐

VITAMINS / SUPPLEMENTS ☐

STEPS: _____

OTHER: _____

Exercise

ACTIVITY	DISTANCE / REPS / TIME

Cardio ☐   Strength ☐

Stretching ☐   Other ☐

Notes

Date

_____

Sleep

7pm · 8 · 9 · 10 · 11 · 12am · 1 · 2 · 3 · 4 · 5 · 6 · 7 · 8 · 9 · 10 · 11 · 12pm

Quality: ☆☆☆☆☆   Hours: _____   Energy Level: ☆☆☆☆☆

Mood

| cheerful | sad | excited | worried | stressed |
| upset | angry | frustrated | content | indifferent |

Meals

BREAKFAST

LUNCH

DINNER

SNACKS

Misc.

WATER: ⬜⬜⬜⬜⬜⬜⬜⬜

VITAMINS / SUPPLEMENTS ⬜

STEPS: _____

OTHER: _____

Exercise

ACTIVITY	DISTANCE / REPS / TIME

Cardio ⬜   Strength ⬜

Stretching ⬜   Other ⬜

Notes

Date

_____

Sunday

Sleep

7pm · 8 · 9 · 10 · 11 · 12am · 1 · 2 · 3 · 4 · 5 · 6 · 7 · 8 · 9 · 10 · 11 · 12pm

Quality: ☆☆☆☆☆   Hours: _____   Energy Level: ☆☆☆☆☆

Mood

| cheerful | sad | excited | worried | stressed |
| upset | angry | frustrated | content | indifferent |

Meals

BREAKFAST

LUNCH

DINNER

SNACKS

Misc.

WATER: ⬜⬜⬜⬜⬜⬜⬜⬜

VITAMINS / SUPPLEMENTS ⬜

STEPS: _____

OTHER: _____

Exercise

ACTIVITY	DISTANCE / REPS / TIME

Cardio ⬜   Strength ⬜

Stretching ⬜   Other ⬜

Notes

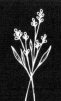 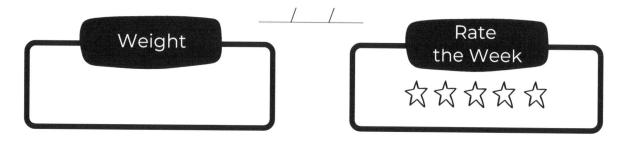 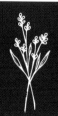

Week 2 Results

_____ / _____ / _____

Weight

Rate the Week

☆☆☆☆☆

What will be the most difficult change you need to make?
What is it so important that you make this change?

_____

_____

_____

_____

What worked well this past week?

_____

_____

_____

What was challenging this past week?

_____

_____

_____

What is one thing you can improve this next week?

_____

_____

_____

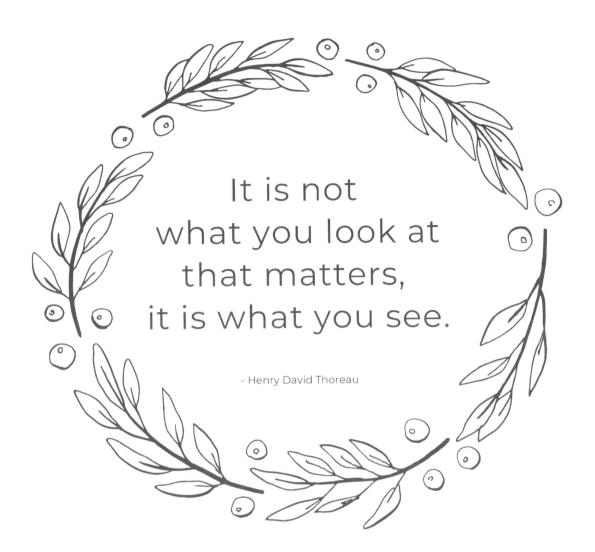

It is not
what you look at
that matters,
it is what you see.

- Henry David Thoreau

MY GOAL FOR THIS WEEK

_____

STEPS I WILL TAKE

_____

_____

_____

Week Three

	Breakfast	Lunch	Dinner	Snacks
Monday				
Tuesday				
Wednesday				
Thursday				
Friday				
Saturday				
Sunday				

Week Three / Meal Plan

Date

_____

Monday

Sleep

7pm · 8 · 9 · 10 · 11 · 12am · 1 · 2 · 3 · 4 · 5 · 6 · 7 · 8 · 9 · 10 · 11 · 12pm

Quality: ☆☆☆☆☆   Hours: _____   Energy Level: ☆☆☆☆☆

Mood

cheerful   sad   excited   worried   stressed

upset   angry   frustrated   content   indifferent

Meals

BREAKFAST
_____
_____
_____
_____

LUNCH
_____
_____
_____

DINNER
_____
_____
_____

SNACKS
_____
_____
_____

Misc.

WATER: ⌷ ⌷ ⌷ ⌷ ⌷ ⌷ ⌷ ⌷

VITAMINS / SUPPLEMENTS ☐

STEPS: _____

OTHER: _____

Exercise

ACTIVITY	DISTANCE / REPS / TIME
_____	_____
_____	_____
_____	_____
_____	_____

Cardio ☐   Strength ☐

Stretching ☐   Other ☐

Notes

_____
_____
_____
_____

Date _____ ~ Tuesday

Sleep

7pm · 8 · 9 · 10 · 11 · 12am · 1 · 2 · 3 · 4 · 5 · 6 · 7 · 8 · 9 · 10 · 11 · 12pm

Quality: ☆☆☆☆☆   Hours: _____   Energy Level: ☆☆☆☆☆

Mood

cheerful	sad	excited	worried	stressed
upset	angry	frustrated	content	indifferent

Meals

BREAKFAST
_____
_____
_____

LUNCH
_____
_____
_____

DINNER
_____
_____
_____

SNACKS
_____
_____

Misc.

WATER: ☐ ☐ ☐ ☐ ☐ ☐ ☐ ☐

VITAMINS / SUPPLEMENTS ☐

STEPS: _____

OTHER: _____

Exercise

ACTIVITY	DISTANCE / REPS / TIME
_____	_____
_____	_____
_____	_____
_____	_____

Cardio ☐   Strength ☐
Stretching ☐   Other ☐

Notes

_____
_____
_____

Date

_____

Wednesday

Sleep

7pm · 8 · 9 · 10 · 11 · 12am · 1 · 2 · 3 · 4 · 5 · 6 · 7 · 8 · 9 · 10 · 11 · 12pm

Quality: ☆☆☆☆☆   Hours: _____   Energy Level: ☆☆☆☆☆

Mood

cheerful   sad   excited   worried   stressed
upset   angry   frustrated   content   indifferent

Meals

BREAKFAST

LUNCH

DINNER

SNACKS

Misc.

WATER: ⬜⬜⬜⬜⬜⬜⬜⬜

VITAMINS / SUPPLEMENTS ☐

STEPS: _____

OTHER: _____

Exercise

ACTIVITY	DISTANCE / REPS / TIME

Cardio ☐   Strength ☐
Stretching ☐   Other ☐

Notes

Date

_____

Sleep

7pm · 8 · 9 · 10 · 11 · 12am · 1 · 2 · 3 · 4 · 5 · 6 · 7 · 8 · 9 · 10 · 11 · 12pm

Quality: ☆☆☆☆☆   Hours: _____   Energy Level: ☆☆☆☆☆

Mood

| cheerful | sad | excited | worried | stressed |
| upset | angry | frustrated | content | indifferent |

Meals

BREAKFAST

LUNCH

DINNER

SNACKS

Misc.

WATER: ⬜⬜⬜⬜⬜⬜⬜⬜

VITAMINS / SUPPLEMENTS ⬜

STEPS: _____

OTHER: _____

Exercise

ACTIVITY	DISTANCE / REPS / TIME

Cardio ⬜   Strength ⬜
Stretching ⬜   Other ⬜

Notes

Date ⟶ _____   Friday

Sleep

7pm · 8 · 9 · 10 · 11 · 12am · 1 · 2 · 3 · 4 · 5 · 6 · 7 · 8 · 9 · 10 · 11 · 12pm

Quality: ☆☆☆☆☆   Hours: _____   Energy Level: ☆☆☆☆☆

Mood

cheerful	sad	excited	worried	stressed
upset	angry	frustrated	content	indifferent

Meals

BREAKFAST
_____
_____
_____

LUNCH
_____
_____
_____

DINNER
_____
_____
_____

SNACKS
_____
_____

Misc.

WATER: ⬜⬜⬜⬜⬜⬜⬜⬜

VITAMINS / SUPPLEMENTS ☐

STEPS: _____

OTHER: _____

Exercise

ACTIVITY	DISTANCE / REPS / TIME
_____	_____
_____	_____
_____	_____

Cardio ☐   Strength ☐
Stretching ☐   Other ☐

Notes

_____
_____
_____

_____

Sleep

7pm · 8 · 9 · 10 · 11 · 12am · 1 · 2 · 3 · 4 · 5 · 6 · 7 · 8 · 9 · 10 · 11 · 12pm

Quality: ☆☆☆☆☆   Hours: _____   Energy Level: ☆☆☆☆☆

Mood

| cheerful | sad | excited | worried | stressed |
| upset | angry | frustrated | content | indifferent |

Meals

BREAKFAST
_____
_____
_____

LUNCH
_____
_____
_____

DINNER
_____
_____
_____

SNACKS
_____
_____

Misc.

WATER: ⬚ ⬚ ⬚ ⬚ ⬚ ⬚ ⬚ ⬚

VITAMINS / SUPPLEMENTS ☐

STEPS: _____

OTHER: _____

Exercise

ACTIVITY	DISTANCE / REPS / TIME
_____	_____
_____	_____
_____	_____
_____	_____

Cardio ☐   Strength ☐

Stretching ☐   Other ☐

Notes

_____
_____
_____

Date

_____

Sunday

Sleep

7pm · 8 · 9 · 10 · 11 · 12am · 1 · 2 · 3 · 4 · 5 · 6 · 7 · 8 · 9 · 10 · 11 · 12pm

Quality: ☆☆☆☆☆   Hours: _____   Energy Level: ☆☆☆☆☆

Mood

cheerful   sad   excited   worried   stressed
upset   angry   frustrated   content   indifferent

Meals

BREAKFAST

LUNCH

DINNER

SNACKS

Misc.

WATER: ⬜⬜⬜⬜⬜⬜⬜⬜

VITAMINS / SUPPLEMENTS ☐

STEPS: _____

OTHER: _____

Exercise

ACTIVITY	DISTANCE / REPS / TIME

Cardio ☐   Strength ☐
Stretching ☐   Other ☐

Notes

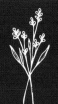 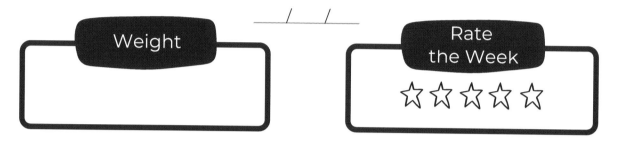 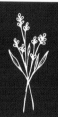

Week 3 Results

_____ / _____ / _____

Weight

Rate the Week
☆ ☆ ☆ ☆ ☆

What emotions drive you toward unhealthy choices?
How can you respond differently to these emotions?

_____
_____
_____
_____

What worked well this past week?

_____
_____
_____

What was challenging this past week?

_____
_____
_____

What is one thing you can improve this next week?

_____
_____
_____

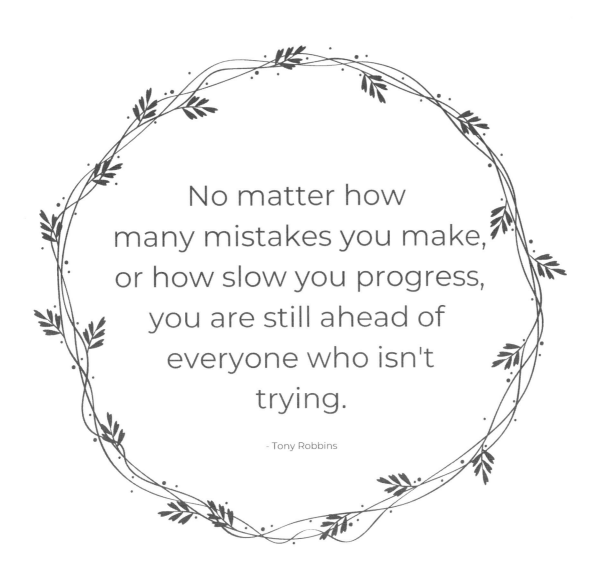

No matter how
many mistakes you make,
or how slow you progress,
you are still ahead of
everyone who isn't
trying.

- Tony Robbins

MY GOAL FOR THIS WEEK

_____

STEPS I WILL TAKE

_____

_____

_____

Week Four

	Breakfast	Lunch	Dinner	Snacks
Monday				
Tuesday				
Wednesday				
Thursday				
Friday				
Saturday				
Sunday				

Week Four / Meal Plan

Date

_____

Monday

Sleep

7pm · 8 · 9 · 10 · 11 · 12am · 1 · 2 · 3 · 4 · 5 · 6 · 7 · 8 · 9 · 10 · 11 · 12pm

Quality: ☆☆☆☆☆   Hours: _____   Energy Level: ☆☆☆☆☆

Mood

| cheerful | sad | excited | worried | stressed |
| upset | angry | frustrated | content | indifferent |

Meals

BREAKFAST

_____
_____
_____
_____

LUNCH

_____
_____
_____

DINNER

_____
_____
_____

SNACKS

_____
_____

Misc.

WATER: ⬜ ⬜ ⬜ ⬜ ⬜ ⬜ ⬜ ⬜

VITAMINS / SUPPLEMENTS ☐

STEPS: _____

OTHER: _____

Exercise

ACTIVITY	DISTANCE / REPS / TIME
_____	_____
_____	_____
_____	_____

Cardio ☐   Strength ☐
Stretching ☐   Other ☐

Notes

_____
_____
_____
_____

Date

Sleep

7pm · 8 · 9 · 10 · 11 · 12am · 1 · 2 · 3 · 4 · 5 · 6 · 7 · 8 · 9 · 10 · 11 · 12pm

Quality: ☆☆☆☆☆   Hours: _____   Energy Level: ☆☆☆☆☆

Mood

| cheerful | sad | excited | worried | stressed |
| upset | angry | frustrated | content | indifferent |

Meals

BREAKFAST

LUNCH

DINNER

SNACKS

Misc.

WATER: ⊓ ⊓ ⊓ ⊓ ⊓ ⊓ ⊓ ⊓

VITAMINS / SUPPLEMENTS ☐

STEPS: _____

OTHER: _____

Exercise

ACTIVITY	DISTANCE / REPS / TIME

Cardio ☐   Strength ☐

Stretching ☐   Other ☐

Notes

Date ❧ Wednesday

_____

Sleep

7pm · 8 · 9 · 10 · 11 · 12am · 1 · 2 · 3 · 4 · 5 · 6 · 7 · 8 · 9 · 10 · 11 · 12pm

Quality: ☆☆☆☆☆   Hours: _____   Energy Level: ☆☆☆☆☆

Mood

cheerful   sad   excited   worried   stressed
upset   angry   frustrated   content   indifferent

Meals

BREAKFAST
_____
_____
_____
_____

LUNCH
_____
_____
_____

DINNER
_____
_____
_____
_____

SNACKS
_____
_____
_____

Misc.

WATER: 🥛🥛🥛🥛🥛🥛🥛🥛

VITAMINS / SUPPLEMENTS ☐

STEPS: _____

OTHER: _____

Exercise

ACTIVITY	DISTANCE / REPS / TIME
_____	_____
_____	_____
_____	_____
_____	_____

Cardio ☐   Strength ☐
Stretching ☐   Other ☐

Notes

_____
_____
_____

Date

Thursday

Sleep

7pm · 8 · 9 · 10 · 11 · 12am · 1 · 2 · 3 · 4 · 5 · 6 · 7 · 8 · 9 · 10 · 11 · 12pm

Quality: ☆☆☆☆☆   Hours: _____   Energy Level: ☆☆☆☆☆

Mood

| cheerful | sad | excited | worried | stressed |
| upset | angry | frustrated | content | indifferent |

Meals

BREAKFAST

LUNCH

DINNER

SNACKS

Misc.

WATER: ▯ ▯ ▯ ▯ ▯ ▯ ▯ ▯

VITAMINS / SUPPLEMENTS ☐

STEPS: _____

OTHER: _____

Exercise

ACTIVITY	DISTANCE / REPS / TIME

Cardio ☐   Strength ☐
Stretching ☐   Other ☐

Notes

Date _____ Friday

Sleep

7pm · 8 · 9 · 10 · 11 · 12am · 1 · 2 · 3 · 4 · 5 · 6 · 7 · 8 · 9 · 10 · 11 · 12pm

Quality: ☆☆☆☆☆   Hours: _____   Energy Level: ☆☆☆☆☆

Mood

cheerful   sad   excited   worried   stressed
upset   angry   frustrated   content   indifferent

Meals

BREAKFAST

LUNCH

DINNER

SNACKS

Misc.

WATER: ⊔⊔⊔⊔⊔⊔⊔⊔

VITAMINS / SUPPLEMENTS ☐

STEPS: _____

OTHER: _____

Exercise

ACTIVITY	DISTANCE / REPS / TIME

Cardio ☐   Strength ☐
Stretching ☐   Other ☐

Notes

Date _____ Saturday

Sleep

7pm · 8 · 9 · 10 · 11 · 12am · 1 · 2 · 3 · 4 · 5 · 6 · 7 · 8 · 9 · 10 · 11 · 12pm

Quality: ☆☆☆☆☆   Hours: _____   Energy Level: ☆☆☆☆☆

Mood

cheerful   sad   excited   worried   stressed
upset   angry   frustrated   content   indifferent

Meals

BREAKFAST

LUNCH

DINNER

SNACKS

Misc.

WATER: ▯ ▯ ▯ ▯ ▯ ▯ ▯ ▯

VITAMINS / SUPPLEMENTS ☐

STEPS: _____

OTHER: _____

Exercise

ACTIVITY	DISTANCE / REPS / TIME

Cardio ☐   Strength ☐
Stretching ☐   Other ☐

Notes

Date

_____

Sunday

Sleep

7pm · 8 · 9 · 10 · 11 · 12am · 1 · 2 · 3 · 4 · 5 · 6 · 7 · 8 · 9 · 10 · 11 · 12pm

Quality: ☆☆☆☆☆   Hours: _____   Energy Level: ☆☆☆☆☆

Mood

| cheerful | sad | excited | worried | stressed |
| upset | angry | frustrated | content | indifferent |

Meals

BREAKFAST

LUNCH

DINNER

SNACKS

Misc.

WATER: ☐ ☐ ☐ ☐ ☐ ☐ ☐ ☐

VITAMINS / SUPPLEMENTS ☐

STEPS: _____

OTHER: _____

Exercise

ACTIVITY	DISTANCE / REPS / TIME

Cardio ☐   Strength ☐

Stretching ☐   Other ☐

Notes

Week 4 Results

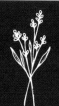
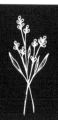

__ / __ / __

Weight

Rate the Week

☆ ☆ ☆ ☆ ☆

What are 1-2 unhealthy items in your pantry or fridge that you need to get rid of right now?

_____

_____

_____

_____

What worked well this past week?

_____

_____

_____

What was challenging this past week?

_____

_____

_____

What is one thing you can improve this next week?

_____

_____

_____

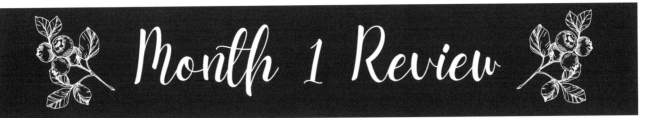

Month 1 Review

Date

Weight

Pounds Lost

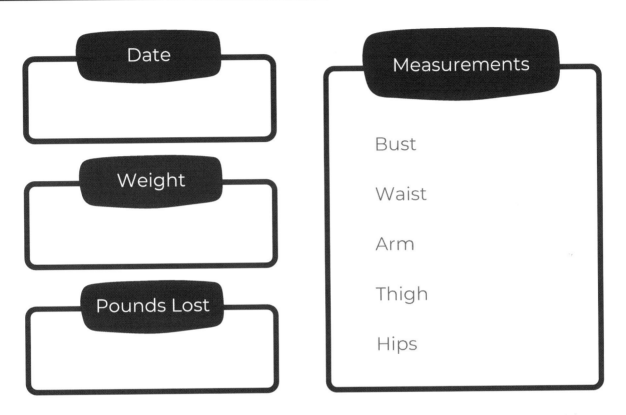

Measurements

Bust

Waist

Arm

Thigh

Hips

List a success or accomplishment you're proud of from this month.

_____

List any old habits that are still a struggle.

_____

_____

_____

List new habits you would like to focus on building next month.

_____

_____

_____

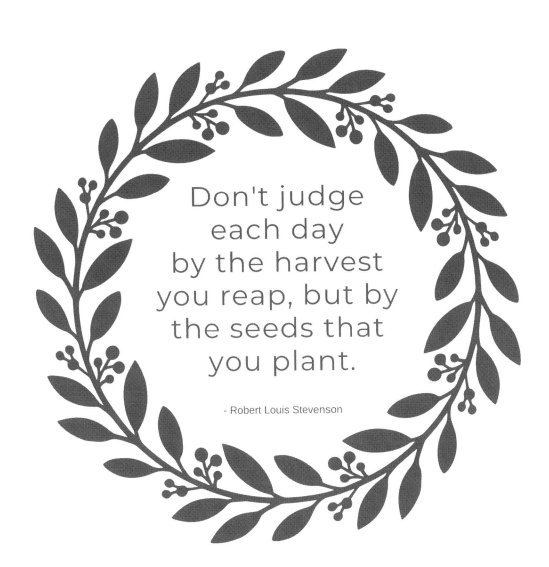

Don't judge
each day
by the harvest
you reap, but by
the seeds that
you plant.

- Robert Louis Stevenson

MY GOAL FOR THIS WEEK

STEPS I WILL TAKE

Week five

	Breakfast	Lunch	Dinner	Snacks
Monday				
Tuesday				
Wednesday				
Thursday				
Friday				
Saturday				
Sunday				

Week Five/ Meal Plan

Date _____

Monday

Sleep

7pm · 8 · 9 · 10 · 11 · 12am · 1 · 2 · 3 · 4 · 5 · 6 · 7 · 8 · 9 · 10 · 11 · 12pm

Quality: ☆☆☆☆☆   Hours: _____   Energy Level: ☆☆☆☆☆

Mood

| cheerful | sad | excited | worried | stressed |
| upset | angry | frustrated | content | indifferent |

Meals

BREAKFAST

LUNCH

DINNER

SNACKS

Misc.

WATER: ▯ ▯ ▯ ▯ ▯ ▯ ▯ ▯

VITAMINS / SUPPLEMENTS ☐

STEPS: _____

OTHER: _____

Exercise

ACTIVITY	DISTANCE / REPS / TIME

Cardio ☐   Strength ☐

Stretching ☐   Other ☐

Notes

Sleep

7pm · 8 · 9 · 10 · 11 · 12am · 1 · 2 · 3 · 4 · 5 · 6 · 7 · 8 · 9 · 10 · 11 · 12pm

Quality: ☆☆☆☆☆   Hours: _____   Energy Level: ☆☆☆☆☆

Mood

| cheerful | sad | excited | worried | stressed |
| upset | angry | frustrated | content | indifferent |

Meals

BREAKFAST
_____
_____
_____
_____

LUNCH
_____
_____
_____
_____

DINNER
_____
_____
_____

SNACKS
_____
_____
_____

Misc.

WATER: ⬜⬜⬜⬜⬜⬜⬜⬜

VITAMINS / SUPPLEMENTS ☐

STEPS: _____

OTHER: _____

Exercise

ACTIVITY	DISTANCE / REPS / TIME
_____	_____
_____	_____
_____	_____
_____	_____

Cardio ☐   Strength ☐
Stretching ☐   Other ☐

Notes

_____
_____
_____

Sleep

7pm · 8 · 9 · 10 · 11 · 12am · 1 · 2 · 3 · 4 · 5 · 6 · 7 · 8 · 9 · 10 · 11 · 12pm

Quality: ☆☆☆☆☆   Hours: _____   Energy Level: ☆☆☆☆☆

Mood

cheerful   sad   excited   worried   stressed
upset   angry   frustrated   content   indifferent

Meals

BREAKFAST

LUNCH

DINNER

SNACKS

Misc.

WATER: ⬜⬜⬜⬜⬜⬜⬜⬜

VITAMINS / SUPPLEMENTS ⬜

STEPS: _____

OTHER: _____

Exercise

ACTIVITY	DISTANCE / REPS / TIME

Cardio ⬜   Strength ⬜
Stretching ⬜   Other ⬜

Notes

Date ~~~~ Thursday

Sleep

7pm · 8 · 9 · 10 · 11 · 12am · 1 · 2 · 3 · 4 · 5 · 6 · 7 · 8 · 9 · 10 · 11 · 12pm

Quality: ☆☆☆☆☆   Hours: _____   Energy Level: ☆☆☆☆☆

Mood

cheerful   sad   excited   worried   stressed
upset   angry   frustrated   content   indifferent

Meals

BREAKFAST
_____
_____
_____

LUNCH
_____
_____
_____

DINNER
_____
_____
_____

SNACKS
_____
_____

Misc.

WATER: ⬛⬛⬛⬛⬛⬛⬛⬛

VITAMINS / SUPPLEMENTS ☐

STEPS: _____

OTHER: _____

Exercise

ACTIVITY	DISTANCE / REPS / TIME
_____	_____
_____	_____
_____	_____
_____	_____

Cardio ☐   Strength ☐
Stretching ☐   Other ☐

Notes

_____
_____
_____

Date _____ Friday

Sleep

7pm · 8 · 9 · 10 · 11 · 12am · 1 · 2 · 3 · 4 · 5 · 6 · 7 · 8 · 9 · 10 · 11 · 12pm

Quality: ☆☆☆☆☆   Hours: _____   Energy Level: ☆☆☆☆☆

Mood

| cheerful | sad | excited | worried | stressed |
| upset | angry | frustrated | content | indifferent |

Meals

BREAKFAST

LUNCH

DINNER

SNACKS

Misc.

WATER: ⛾ ⛾ ⛾ ⛾ ⛾ ⛾ ⛾ ⛾

VITAMINS / SUPPLEMENTS ☐

STEPS: _____

OTHER: _____

Exercise

ACTIVITY	DISTANCE / REPS / TIME

Cardio ☐   Strength ☐

Stretching ☐   Other ☐

Notes

Date _____   ## Saturday

Sleep

7pm · 8 · 9 · 10 · 11 · 12am · 1 · 2 · 3 · 4 · 5 · 6 · 7 · 8 · 9 · 10 · 11 · 12pm

Quality: ☆☆☆☆☆   Hours: _____   Energy Level: ☆☆☆☆☆

Mood

cheerful	sad	excited	worried	stressed
upset	angry	frustrated	content	indifferent

Meals

BREAKFAST
_____
_____
_____
_____

LUNCH
_____
_____
_____
_____

DINNER
_____
_____
_____
_____

SNACKS
_____
_____
_____

Misc.

WATER: ☐ ☐ ☐ ☐ ☐ ☐ ☐ ☐

VITAMINS / SUPPLEMENTS ☐

STEPS: _____

OTHER: _____

Exercise

ACTIVITY	DISTANCE / REPS / TIME
_____	_____
_____	_____
_____	_____

Cardio ☐   Strength ☐
Stretching ☐   Other ☐

Notes

_____
_____
_____

Sleep

7pm · 8 · 9 · 10 · 11 · 12am · 1 · 2 · 3 · 4 · 5 · 6 · 7 · 8 · 9 · 10 · 11 · 12pm

Quality: ☆☆☆☆☆   Hours: _____   Energy Level: ☆☆☆☆☆

Mood

| cheerful | sad | excited | worried | stressed |
| upset | angry | frustrated | content | indifferent |

Meals

BREAKFAST

LUNCH

DINNER

SNACKS

Misc.

WATER: ⬜⬜⬜⬜⬜⬜⬜⬜

VITAMINS / SUPPLEMENTS ⬜

STEPS: _____

OTHER: _____

Exercise

ACTIVITY	DISTANCE / REPS / TIME

Cardio ⬜   Strength ⬜
Stretching ⬜   Other ⬜

Notes

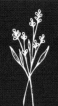 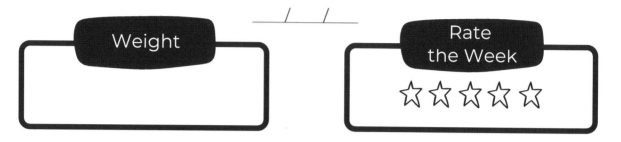 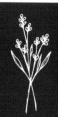

Week 5 Results

_____ / _____ / _____

Weight

Rate the Week

☆ ☆ ☆ ☆ ☆

List 3-4 adjectives that describe how you feel about exercise.
How can you redefine exercise in your life so it's a pleasant experience?

_____

_____

_____

_____

What worked well this past week?

_____

_____

_____

What was challenging this past week?

_____

_____

_____

What is one thing you can improve this next week?

_____

_____

_____

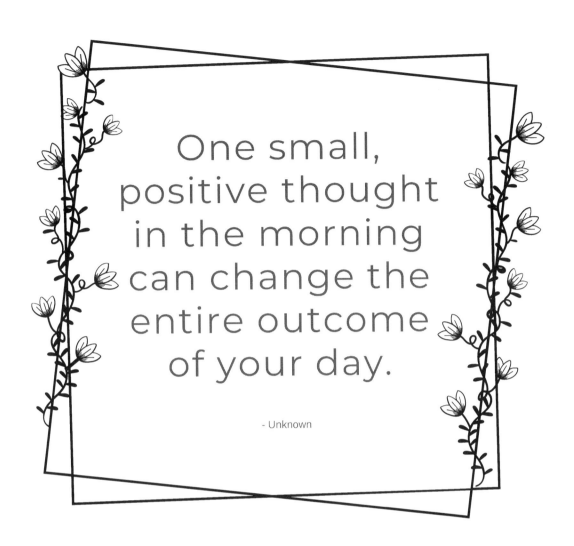

One small,
positive thought
in the morning
can change the
entire outcome
of your day.

- Unknown

MY GOAL FOR THIS WEEK

_____

STEPS I WILL TAKE

_____

_____

_____

Week Six

	Breakfast	Lunch	Dinner	Snacks
Monday				
Tuesday				
Wednesday				
Thursday				
Friday				
Saturday				
Sunday				

Week Six / Meal Plan

Date

Monday

Sleep

7pm · 8 · 9 · 10 · 11 · 12am · 1 · 2 · 3 · 4 · 5 · 6 · 7 · 8 · 9 · 10 · 11 · 12pm

Quality: ☆☆☆☆☆   Hours: _____   Energy Level: ☆☆☆☆☆

Mood

| cheerful | sad | excited | worried | stressed |
| upset | angry | frustrated | content | indifferent |

Meals

BREAKFAST

LUNCH

DINNER

SNACKS

Misc.

WATER: ▯ ▯ ▯ ▯ ▯ ▯ ▯ ▯

VITAMINS / SUPPLEMENTS ☐

STEPS: _____

OTHER: _____

Exercise

| ACTIVITY | DISTANCE / REPS / TIME |

Cardio ☐   Strength ☐

Stretching ☐   Other ☐

Notes

Date _____ Tuesday

Sleep

7pm · 8 · 9 · 10 · 11 · 12am · 1 · 2 · 3 · 4 · 5 · 6 · 7 · 8 · 9 · 10 · 11 · 12pm

Quality: ☆ ☆ ☆ ☆ ☆   Hours: _____   Energy Level: ☆ ☆ ☆ ☆ ☆

Mood

cheerful   sad   excited   worried   stressed

upset   angry   frustrated   content   indifferent

Meals

BREAKFAST

LUNCH

DINNER

SNACKS

Misc.

WATER: ⌷ ⌷ ⌷ ⌷ ⌷ ⌷ ⌷ ⌷

VITAMINS / SUPPLEMENTS ☐

STEPS: _____

OTHER: _____

Exercise

ACTIVITY	DISTANCE / REPS / TIME

Cardio ☐   Strength ☐

Stretching ☐   Other ☐

Notes

Sleep

7pm · 8 · 9 · 10 · 11 · 12am · 1 · 2 · 3 · 4 · 5 · 6 · 7 · 8 · 9 · 10 · 11 · 12pm

Quality: ☆☆☆☆☆   Hours: _____   Energy Level: ☆☆☆☆☆

Mood

| cheerful | sad | excited | worried | stressed |
| upset | angry | frustrated | content | indifferent |

Meals

BREAKFAST
_____
_____
_____

LUNCH
_____
_____
_____

DINNER
_____
_____
_____

SNACKS
_____
_____

Misc.

WATER: ▯ ▯ ▯ ▯ ▯ ▯ ▯ ▯

VITAMINS / SUPPLEMENTS ☐

STEPS: _____

OTHER: _____

Exercise

ACTIVITY	DISTANCE / REPS / TIME
_____	_____
_____	_____
_____	_____
_____	_____

Cardio ☐   Strength ☐
Stretching ☐   Other ☐

Notes

_____
_____
_____

Date

Thursday

Sleep

7pm · 8 · 9 · 10 · 11 · 12am · 1 · 2 · 3 · 4 · 5 · 6 · 7 · 8 · 9 · 10 · 11 · 12pm

Quality: ☆☆☆☆☆   Hours: _____   Energy Level: ☆☆☆☆☆

Mood

cheerful	sad	excited	worried	stressed
upset	angry	frustrated	content	indifferent

Meals

BREAKFAST
_____
_____
_____

LUNCH
_____
_____
_____

DINNER
_____
_____
_____

SNACKS
_____
_____

Misc.

WATER: ⬜⬜⬜⬜⬜⬜⬜⬜

VITAMINS / SUPPLEMENTS ☐

STEPS: _____

OTHER: _____

Exercise

ACTIVITY	DISTANCE / REPS / TIME

Cardio ☐   Strength ☐
Stretching ☐   Other ☐

Notes

_____
_____
_____

Date

Sleep

7pm · 8 · 9 · 10 · 11 · 12am · 1 · 2 · 3 · 4 · 5 · 6 · 7 · 8 · 9 · 10 · 11 · 12pm

Quality: ☆☆☆☆☆   Hours: _____   Energy Level: ☆☆☆☆☆

Mood

cheerful   sad   excited   worried   stressed
upset   angry   frustrated   content   indifferent

Meals

BREAKFAST

LUNCH

DINNER

SNACKS

Misc.

WATER: ⬜⬜⬜⬜⬜⬜⬜⬜

VITAMINS / SUPPLEMENTS ☐

STEPS: _____

OTHER: _____

Exercise

ACTIVITY	DISTANCE / REPS / TIME

Cardio ☐   Strength ☐
Stretching ☐   Other ☐

Notes

Sleep

7pm · 8 · 9 · 10 · 11 · 12am · 1 · 2 · 3 · 4 · 5 · 6 · 7 · 8 · 9 · 10 · 11 · 12pm

Quality: ☆☆☆☆☆   Hours: _____   Energy Level: ☆☆☆☆☆

Mood

cheerful   sad   excited   worried   stressed
upset   angry   frustrated   content   indifferent

Meals

BREAKFAST
_____
_____
_____

LUNCH
_____
_____
_____

DINNER
_____
_____
_____

SNACKS
_____
_____

Misc.

WATER: ⊓ ⊓ ⊓ ⊓ ⊓ ⊓ ⊓ ⊓

VITAMINS / SUPPLEMENTS ☐

STEPS: _____

OTHER: _____

Exercise

ACTIVITY	DISTANCE / REPS / TIME
_____	_____
_____	_____
_____	_____
_____	_____

Cardio ☐   Strength ☐
Stretching ☐   Other ☐

Notes

_____
_____
_____

Date _____

Sunday

Sleep

7pm · 8 · 9 · 10 · 11 · 12am · 1 · 2 · 3 · 4 · 5 · 6 · 7 · 8 · 9 · 10 · 11 · 12pm

Quality: ☆☆☆☆☆   Hours: _____   Energy Level: ☆☆☆☆☆

Mood

| cheerful | sad | excited | worried | stressed |
| upset | angry | frustrated | content | indifferent |

Meals

BREAKFAST

LUNCH

DINNER

SNACKS

Misc.

WATER: ⬚ ⬚ ⬚ ⬚ ⬚ ⬚ ⬚ ⬚

VITAMINS / SUPPLEMENTS ☐

STEPS: _____

OTHER: _____

Exercise

ACTIVITY	DISTANCE / REPS / TIME

Cardio ☐   Strength ☐
Stretching ☐   Other ☐

Notes

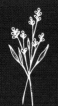 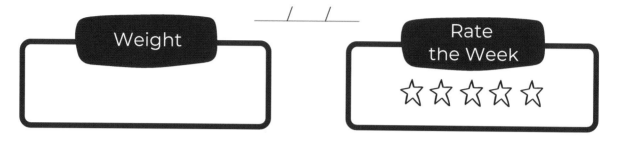 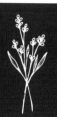

Week 6 Results

_____ / _____ / _____

Weight

Rate the Week

☆ ☆ ☆ ☆ ☆

What are 2-3 changes you can make to your environment
to support your healthy lifestyle?

_____

_____

_____

_____

What worked well this past week?

_____

_____

_____

What was challenging this past week?

_____

_____

_____

What is one thing you can improve this next week?

_____

_____

_____

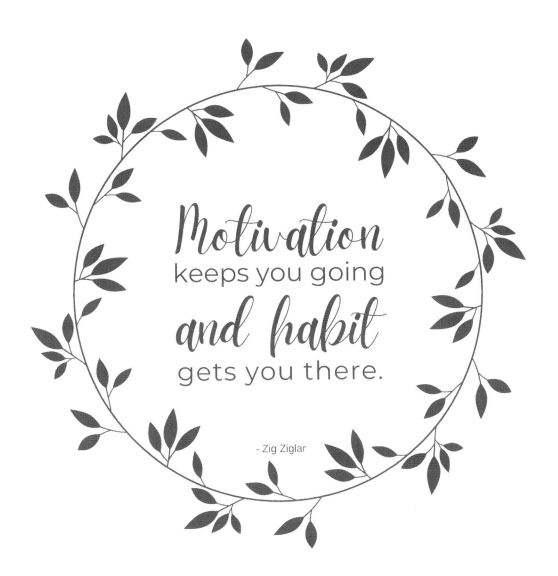

Motivation keeps you going *and habit* gets you there.

- Zig Ziglar

MY GOAL FOR THIS WEEK

_____

STEPS I WILL TAKE

_____

_____

_____

Week Seven

	Breakfast	Lunch	Dinner	Snacks
Monday				
Tuesday				
Wednesday				
Thursday				
Friday				
Saturday				
Sunday				

Week Seven / Meal Plan

Date

_____

Sleep

7pm · 8 · 9 · 10 · 11 · 12am · 1 · 2 · 3 · 4 · 5 · 6 · 7 · 8 · 9 · 10 · 11 · 12pm

Quality: ☆☆☆☆☆   Hours: _____   Energy Level: ☆☆☆☆☆

Mood

| cheerful | sad | excited | worried | stressed |
| upset | angry | frustrated | content | indifferent |

Meals

BREAKFAST
_____
_____
_____
_____

LUNCH
_____
_____
_____
_____

DINNER
_____
_____
_____
_____

SNACKS
_____
_____
_____

Misc.

WATER: ⬜⬜⬜⬜⬜⬜⬜⬜

VITAMINS / SUPPLEMENTS ☐

STEPS: _____

OTHER: _____

Exercise

ACTIVITY	DISTANCE / REPS / TIME
_____	_____
_____	_____
_____	_____
_____	_____

Cardio ☐   Strength ☐
Stretching ☐   Other ☐

Notes

_____
_____
_____

Date

_____

Sleep

7pm · 8 · 9 · 10 · 11 · 12am · 1 · 2 · 3 · 4 · 5 · 6 · 7 · 8 · 9 · 10 · 11 · 12pm

Quality: ☆☆☆☆☆   Hours: _____   Energy Level: ☆☆☆☆☆

Mood

cheerful   sad   excited   worried   stressed
upset   angry   frustrated   content   indifferent

Meals

BREAKFAST
_____
_____
_____
_____

LUNCH
_____
_____
_____
_____

DINNER
_____
_____
_____
_____

SNACKS
_____
_____
_____

Misc.

WATER: ⬜⬜⬜⬜⬜⬜⬜⬜

VITAMINS / SUPPLEMENTS ☐

STEPS: _____

OTHER: _____

Exercise

ACTIVITY	DISTANCE / REPS / TIME
_____	_____
_____	_____
_____	_____
_____	_____

Cardio ☐   Strength ☐
Stretching ☐   Other ☐

Notes

_____
_____
_____

Date

_____

Sleep

7pm · 8 · 9 · 10 · 11 · 12am · 1 · 2 · 3 · 4 · 5 · 6 · 7 · 8 · 9 · 10 · 11 · 12pm

Quality: ☆☆☆☆☆   Hours: _____   Energy Level: ☆☆☆☆☆

Mood

cheerful   sad   excited   worried   stressed
upset   angry   frustrated   content   indifferent

Meals

BREAKFAST

LUNCH

DINNER

SNACKS

Misc.

WATER: 🥛🥛🥛🥛🥛🥛🥛🥛

VITAMINS / SUPPLEMENTS ☐

STEPS: _____

OTHER: _____

Exercise

ACTIVITY	DISTANCE / REPS / TIME

Cardio ☐   Strength ☐
Stretching ☐   Other ☐

Notes

Date _____   Thursday

Sleep

7pm · 8 · 9 · 10 · 11 · 12am · 1 · 2 · 3 · 4 · 5 · 6 · 7 · 8 · 9 · 10 · 11 · 12pm

Quality: ☆☆☆☆☆   Hours: _____   Energy Level: ☆☆☆☆☆

Mood

| cheerful | sad | excited | worried | stressed |
| upset | angry | frustrated | content | indifferent |

Meals

BREAKFAST

LUNCH

DINNER

SNACKS

Misc.

WATER: ⬜⬜⬜⬜⬜⬜⬜⬜

VITAMINS / SUPPLEMENTS ☐

STEPS: _____

OTHER: _____

Exercise

ACTIVITY	DISTANCE / REPS / TIME

Cardio ☐   Strength ☐
Stretching ☐   Other ☐

Notes

Date

Friday

_____

Sleep

7pm · 8 · 9 · 10 · 11 · 12am · 1 · 2 · 3 · 4 · 5 · 6 · 7 · 8 · 9 · 10 · 11 · 12pm

Quality: ☆☆☆☆☆   Hours: _____   Energy Level: ☆☆☆☆☆

Mood

| cheerful | sad | excited | worried | stressed |
| upset | angry | frustrated | content | indifferent |

Meals

BREAKFAST

LUNCH

DINNER

SNACKS

Misc.

WATER: ⬜⬜⬜⬜⬜⬜⬜⬜

VITAMINS / SUPPLEMENTS ☐

STEPS: _____

OTHER: _____

Exercise

ACTIVITY	DISTANCE / REPS / TIME

Cardio ☐   Strength ☐

Stretching ☐   Other ☐

Notes

Date

Saturday

_____

Sleep

7pm · 8 · 9 · 10 · 11 · 12am · 1 · 2 · 3 · 4 · 5 · 6 · 7 · 8 · 9 · 10 · 11 · 12pm

Quality: ☆☆☆☆☆   Hours: _____   Energy Level: ☆☆☆☆☆

Mood

cheerful	sad	excited	worried	stressed
upset	angry	frustrated	content	indifferent

Meals

BREAKFAST
_____
_____
_____

LUNCH
_____
_____
_____

DINNER
_____
_____
_____

SNACKS
_____
_____
_____

Misc.

WATER: 🥛🥛🥛🥛🥛🥛🥛🥛

VITAMINS / SUPPLEMENTS ☐

STEPS: _____

OTHER: _____

Exercise

ACTIVITY	DISTANCE / REPS / TIME
_____	_____
_____	_____
_____	_____

Cardio ☐   Strength ☐

Stretching ☐   Other ☐

Notes

_____
_____
_____

Sleep

7pm · 8 · 9 · 10 · 11 · 12am · 1 · 2 · 3 · 4 · 5 · 6 · 7 · 8 · 9 · 10 · 11 · 12pm

Quality: ☆☆☆☆☆   Hours: _____   Energy Level: ☆☆☆☆☆

Mood

| cheerful | sad | excited | worried | stressed |
| upset | angry | frustrated | content | indifferent |

Meals

BREAKFAST
_____
_____
_____
_____

LUNCH
_____
_____
_____

DINNER
_____
_____
_____

SNACKS
_____
_____
_____

Misc.

WATER: ☐ ☐ ☐ ☐ ☐ ☐ ☐ ☐

VITAMINS / SUPPLEMENTS ☐

STEPS: _____

OTHER: _____

Exercise

ACTIVITY	DISTANCE / REPS / TIME
_____	_____
_____	_____
_____	_____

Cardio ☐   Strength ☐
Stretching ☐   Other ☐

Notes

_____
_____
_____
_____

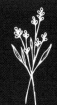 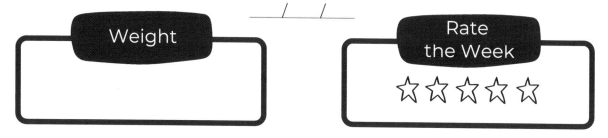 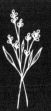

Week 7 Results

_____ / ____ / ____

Weight

Rate the Week
☆ ☆ ☆ ☆ ☆

List 2-3 activities you enjoy that require moving your body regularly.
How can you do these activities more often?

_____

_____

_____

_____

What worked well this past week?

_____

_____

_____

What was challenging this past week?

_____

_____

_____

What is one thing you can improve this next week?

_____

_____

_____

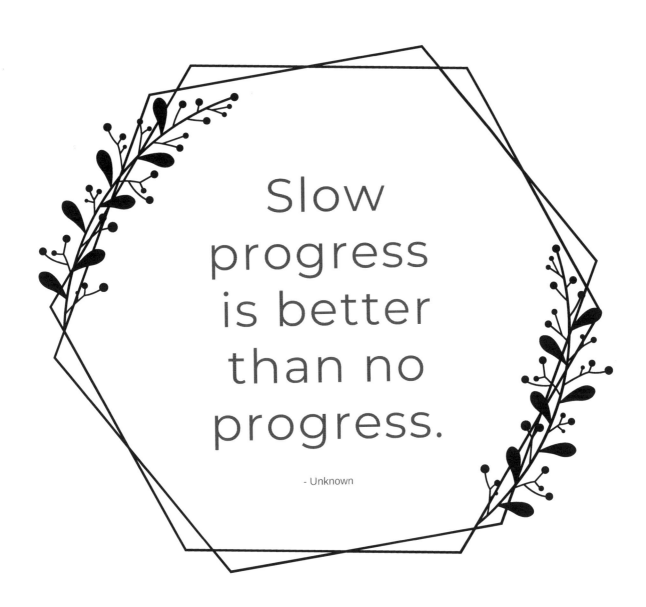

Slow
progress
is better
than no
progress.

- Unknown

MY GOAL FOR THIS WEEK

_____

STEPS I WILL TAKE

_____

_____

_____

Week Eight

	Breakfast	Lunch	Dinner	Snacks
Monday				
Tuesday				
Wednesday				
Thursday				
Friday				
Saturday				
Sunday				

Week Eight / Meal Plan

Date

Monday

Sleep

7pm · 8 · 9 · 10 · 11 · 12am · 1 · 2 · 3 · 4 · 5 · 6 · 7 · 8 · 9 · 10 · 11 · 12pm

Quality: ☆☆☆☆☆   Hours: _____   Energy Level: ☆☆☆☆☆

Mood

| cheerful | sad | excited | worried | stressed |
| upset | angry | frustrated | content | indifferent |

Meals

BREAKFAST
_____
_____
_____
_____

LUNCH
_____
_____
_____
_____

DINNER
_____
_____
_____
_____

SNACKS
_____
_____
_____

Misc.

WATER: ⊔ ⊔ ⊔ ⊔ ⊔ ⊔ ⊔ ⊔

VITAMINS / SUPPLEMENTS ☐

STEPS: _____

OTHER: _____

Exercise

ACTIVITY	DISTANCE / REPS / TIME
_____	_____
_____	_____
_____	_____

Cardio ☐   Strength ☐
Stretching ☐   Other ☐

Notes

_____
_____
_____

Sleep

7pm · 8 · 9 · 10 · 11 · 12am · 1 · 2 · 3 · 4 · 5 · 6 · 7 · 8 · 9 · 10 · 11 · 12pm

Quality: ☆☆☆☆☆   Hours: _____   Energy Level: ☆☆☆☆☆

Mood

| cheerful | sad | excited | worried | stressed |
| upset | angry | frustrated | content | indifferent |

Meals

BREAKFAST
_____
_____
_____
_____

LUNCH
_____
_____
_____
_____

DINNER
_____
_____
_____
_____

SNACKS
_____
_____
_____

Misc.

WATER: 🥛🥛🥛🥛🥛🥛🥛🥛

VITAMINS / SUPPLEMENTS ☐

STEPS: _____

OTHER: _____

Exercise

ACTIVITY	DISTANCE / REPS / TIME
_____	_____
_____	_____
_____	_____
_____	_____

Cardio ☐   Strength ☐
Stretching ☐   Other ☐

Notes

_____
_____
_____

Date

_____

Sleep

7pm · 8 · 9 · 10 · 11 · 12am · 1 · 2 · 3 · 4 · 5 · 6 · 7 · 8 · 9 · 10 · 11 · 12pm

Quality: ☆☆☆☆☆   Hours: _____   Energy Level: ☆☆☆☆☆

Wednesday

Mood

| cheerful | sad | excited | worried | stressed |
| upset | angry | frustrated | content | indifferent |

Meals

BREAKFAST

_____
_____
_____
_____

LUNCH

_____
_____
_____
_____

DINNER

_____
_____
_____
_____

SNACKS

_____
_____
_____

Misc.

WATER: ☐ ☐ ☐ ☐ ☐ ☐ ☐ ☐

VITAMINS / SUPPLEMENTS ☐

STEPS: _____

OTHER: _____

Exercise

ACTIVITY	DISTANCE / REPS / TIME
_____	_____
_____	_____
_____	_____

Cardio ☐   Strength ☐
Stretching ☐   Other ☐

Notes

_____
_____
_____

Sleep

7pm · 8 · 9 · 10 · 11 · 12am · 1 · 2 · 3 · 4 · 5 · 6 · 7 · 8 · 9 · 10 · 11 · 12pm

Quality: ☆ ☆ ☆ ☆ ☆   Hours: _____   Energy Level: ☆ ☆ ☆ ☆ ☆

Mood

| cheerful | sad | excited | worried | stressed |
| upset | angry | frustrated | content | indifferent |

Meals

BREAKFAST
_____
_____
_____

LUNCH
_____
_____
_____

DINNER
_____
_____
_____

SNACKS
_____
_____

Misc.

WATER: ▯ ▯ ▯ ▯ ▯ ▯ ▯ ▯

VITAMINS / SUPPLEMENTS ☐

STEPS: _____

OTHER: _____

Exercise

ACTIVITY	DISTANCE / REPS / TIME
_____	_____
_____	_____
_____	_____
_____	_____

Cardio ☐   Strength ☐
Stretching ☐   Other ☐

Notes

_____
_____
_____

Sleep

7pm · 8 · 9 · 10 · 11 · 12am · 1 · 2 · 3 · 4 · 5 · 6 · 7 · 8 · 9 · 10 · 11 · 12pm

Quality: ☆ ☆ ☆ ☆ ☆   Hours: _____   Energy Level: ☆ ☆ ☆ ☆ ☆

Mood

| cheerful | sad | excited | worried | stressed |
| upset | angry | frustrated | content | indifferent |

Meals

BREAKFAST

LUNCH

DINNER

SNACKS

Misc.

WATER: ⬜ ⬜ ⬜ ⬜ ⬜ ⬜ ⬜ ⬜

VITAMINS / SUPPLEMENTS ☐

STEPS: _____

OTHER: _____

Exercise

ACTIVITY	DISTANCE / REPS / TIME

Cardio ☐   Strength ☐

Stretching ☐   Other ☐

Notes

Sleep

7pm · 8 · 9 · 10 · 11 · 12am · 1 · 2 · 3 · 4 · 5 · 6 · 7 · 8 · 9 · 10 · 11 · 12pm

Quality: ☆☆☆☆☆   Hours: _____   Energy Level: ☆☆☆☆☆

Mood

| cheerful | sad | excited | worried | stressed |
| upset | angry | frustrated | content | indifferent |

Meals

BREAKFAST

LUNCH

DINNER

SNACKS

Misc.

WATER: 🥤 🥤 🥤 🥤 🥤 🥤 🥤 🥤

VITAMINS / SUPPLEMENTS ☐

STEPS: _____

OTHER: _____

Exercise

ACTIVITY	DISTANCE / REPS / TIME

Cardio ☐   Strength ☐
Stretching ☐   Other ☐

Notes

Date
Sunday

_____

Sleep

7pm · 8 · 9 · 10 · 11 · 12am · 1 · 2 · 3 · 4 · 5 · 6 · 7 · 8 · 9 · 10 · 11 · 12pm

Quality: ☆ ☆ ☆ ☆ ☆   Hours: _____   Energy Level: ☆ ☆ ☆ ☆ ☆

Mood

| cheerful | sad | excited | worried | stressed |
| upset | angry | frustrated | content | indifferent |

Meals

BREAKFAST
_____
_____
_____
_____

LUNCH
_____
_____
_____
_____

DINNER
_____
_____
_____
_____

SNACKS
_____
_____
_____

Misc.

WATER: ▯ ▯ ▯ ▯ ▯ ▯ ▯ ▯

VITAMINS / SUPPLEMENTS ☐

STEPS: _____

OTHER: _____

Exercise

ACTIVITY	DISTANCE / REPS / TIME
_____	_____
_____	_____
_____	_____
_____	_____

Cardio ☐   Strength ☐
Stretching ☐   Other ☐

Notes

_____
_____
_____

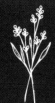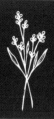

Week 8 Results

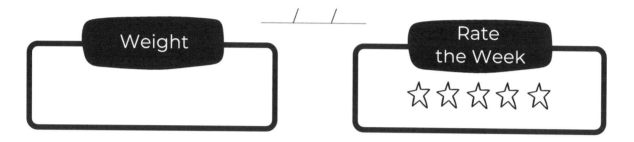

/ /

Weight

Rate the Week
☆ ☆ ☆ ☆ ☆

What attitude do you need to cultivate when you experience setbacks?
How will this help you stay focused on succeeding?

_____
_____
_____
_____

What worked well this past week?

_____
_____
_____

What was challenging this past week?

_____
_____
_____

What is one thing you can improve this next week?

_____
_____
_____

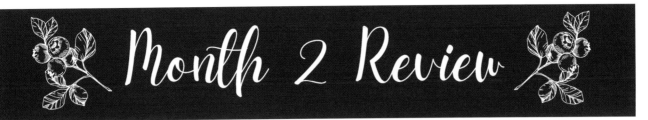

Month 2 Review

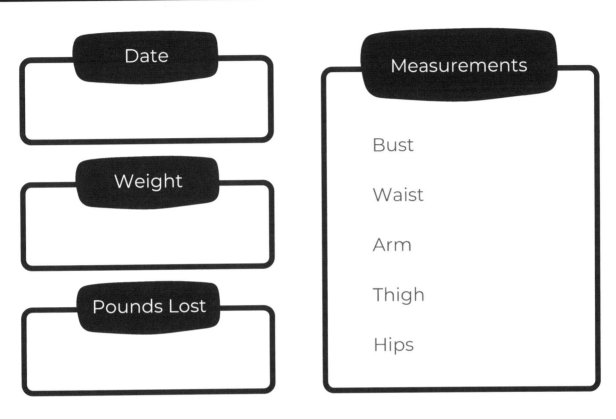

Date

Weight

Pounds Lost

Measurements

Bust

Waist

Arm

Thigh

Hips

List a success or accomplishment you're proud of from this month.

_____

List any old habits that are still a struggle.

_____

_____

_____

List new habits you would like to focus on building next month.

_____

_____

_____

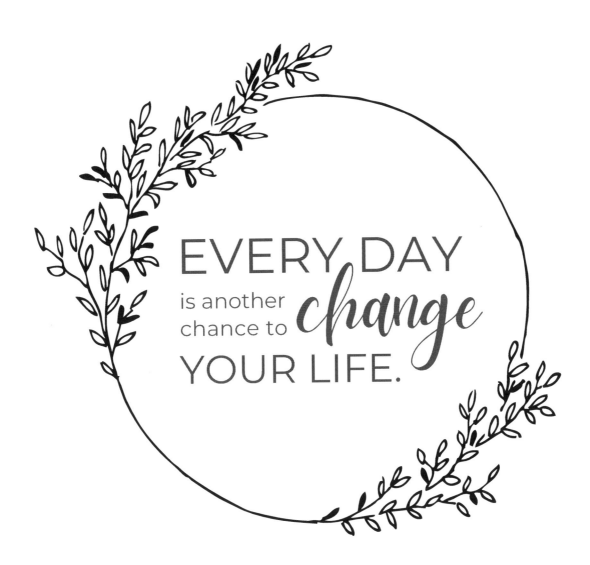

EVERY DAY
is another chance to *change*
YOUR LIFE.

MY GOAL FOR THIS WEEK

_____

STEPS I WILL TAKE

_____

_____

_____

Week Nine

	Breakfast	Lunch	Dinner	Snacks
Monday				
Tuesday				
Wednesday				
Thursday				
Friday				
Saturday				
Sunday				

Week Nine / Meal Plan

Date

_____

Monday

Sleep

7pm · 8 · 9 · 10 · 11 · 12am · 1 · 2 · 3 · 4 · 5 · 6 · 7 · 8 · 9 · 10 · 11 · 12pm

Quality: ☆☆☆☆☆   Hours: _____   Energy Level: ☆☆☆☆☆

Mood

cheerful	sad	excited	worried	stressed
upset	angry	frustrated	content	indifferent

Meals

BREAKFAST
_____
_____
_____
_____

LUNCH
_____
_____
_____
_____

DINNER
_____
_____
_____
_____

SNACKS
_____
_____
_____

Misc.

WATER: ⬜⬜⬜⬜⬜⬜⬜⬜

VITAMINS / SUPPLEMENTS ⬜

STEPS: _____

OTHER: _____

Exercise

ACTIVITY	DISTANCE / REPS / TIME

Cardio ⬜   Strength ⬜
Stretching ⬜   Other ⬜

Notes

_____
_____
_____

Date _____ Tuesday

Sleep

7pm · 8 · 9 · 10 · 11 · 12am · 1 · 2 · 3 · 4 · 5 · 6 · 7 · 8 · 9 · 10 · 11 · 12pm

Quality: ☆☆☆☆☆   Hours: _____   Energy Level: ☆☆☆☆☆

Mood

cheerful   sad   excited   worried   stressed
upset   angry   frustrated   content   indifferent

Meals

BREAKFAST
_____
_____
_____

LUNCH
_____
_____
_____

DINNER
_____
_____
_____

SNACKS
_____
_____

Misc.

WATER: ⬚⬚⬚⬚⬚⬚⬚⬚

VITAMINS / SUPPLEMENTS ☐

STEPS: _____

OTHER: _____

Exercise

ACTIVITY	DISTANCE / REPS / TIME
_____	_____
_____	_____
_____	_____
_____	_____

Cardio ☐   Strength ☐
Stretching ☐   Other ☐

Notes

_____
_____
_____

_____

Sleep

7pm · 8 · 9 · 10 · 11 · 12am · 1 · 2 · 3 · 4 · 5 · 6 · 7 · 8 · 9 · 10 · 11 · 12pm

Quality: ☆☆☆☆☆   Hours: _____   Energy Level: ☆☆☆☆☆

Mood

| cheerful | sad | excited | worried | stressed |
| upset | angry | frustrated | content | indifferent |

Meals

BREAKFAST
_____
_____
_____
_____

LUNCH
_____
_____
_____
_____

DINNER
_____
_____
_____
_____

SNACKS
_____
_____
_____

Misc.

WATER: ⬜⬜⬜⬜⬜⬜⬜⬜

VITAMINS / SUPPLEMENTS ☐

STEPS: _____

OTHER: _____

Exercise

ACTIVITY	DISTANCE / REPS / TIME
_____	_____
_____	_____
_____	_____
_____	_____

Cardio ☐   Strength ☐
Stretching ☐   Other ☐

Notes

_____
_____
_____

Date

_____

Sleep

7pm · 8 · 9 · 10 · 11 · 12am · 1 · 2 · 3 · 4 · 5 · 6 · 7 · 8 · 9 · 10 · 11 · 12pm

Quality: ☆☆☆☆☆   Hours: _____   Energy Level: ☆☆☆☆☆

Mood

cheerful   sad   excited   worried   stressed
upset   angry   frustrated   content   indifferent

Meals

BREAKFAST
_____
_____
_____
_____

LUNCH
_____
_____
_____
_____

DINNER
_____
_____
_____
_____

SNACKS
_____
_____
_____

Misc.

WATER: ☐ ☐ ☐ ☐ ☐ ☐ ☐ ☐

VITAMINS / SUPPLEMENTS ☐

STEPS: _____

OTHER: _____

Exercise

ACTIVITY	DISTANCE / REPS / TIME
_____	_____
_____	_____
_____	_____
_____	_____

Cardio ☐   Strength ☐
Stretching ☐   Other ☐

Notes

_____
_____
_____
_____

Date

_____

Sleep

7pm · 8 · 9 · 10 · 11 · 12am · 1 · 2 · 3 · 4 · 5 · 6 · 7 · 8 · 9 · 10 · 11 · 12pm

Quality: ☆☆☆☆☆   Hours: _____   Energy Level: ☆☆☆☆☆

Mood

| cheerful | sad | excited | worried | stressed |
| upset | angry | frustrated | content | indifferent |

Meals

BREAKFAST

LUNCH

DINNER

SNACKS

Misc.

WATER: ⬛⬛⬛⬛⬛⬛⬛⬛

VITAMINS / SUPPLEMENTS ☐

STEPS: _____

OTHER: _____

Exercise

ACTIVITY	DISTANCE / REPS / TIME

Cardio ☐   Strength ☐

Stretching ☐   Other ☐

Notes

Date

Saturday

Sleep

7pm · 8 · 9 · 10 · 11 · 12am · 1 · 2 · 3 · 4 · 5 · 6 · 7 · 8 · 9 · 10 · 11 · 12pm

Quality: ☆☆☆☆☆   Hours: _____   Energy Level: ☆☆☆☆☆

Mood

| cheerful | sad | excited | worried | stressed |
| upset | angry | frustrated | content | indifferent |

Meals

BREAKFAST

LUNCH

DINNER

SNACKS

Misc.

WATER: 🥛🥛🥛🥛🥛🥛🥛🥛

VITAMINS / SUPPLEMENTS ☐

STEPS: _____

OTHER: _____

Exercise

| ACTIVITY | DISTANCE / REPS / TIME |

Cardio ☐   Strength ☐
Stretching ☐   Other ☐

Notes

Sleep

7pm · 8 · 9 · 10 · 11 · 12am · 1 · 2 · 3 · 4 · 5 · 6 · 7 · 8 · 9 · 10 · 11 · 12pm

Quality: ☆ ☆ ☆ ☆ ☆   Hours: _____   Energy Level: ☆ ☆ ☆ ☆ ☆

Mood

| cheerful | sad | excited | worried | stressed |
| upset | angry | frustrated | content | indifferent |

Meals

BREAKFAST
_____
_____
_____
_____

LUNCH
_____
_____
_____
_____

DINNER
_____
_____
_____
_____

SNACKS
_____
_____
_____

Misc.

WATER: ⬜ ⬜ ⬜ ⬜ ⬜ ⬜ ⬜ ⬜

VITAMINS / SUPPLEMENTS ☐

STEPS: _____

OTHER: _____

Exercise

ACTIVITY	DISTANCE / REPS / TIME
_____	_____
_____	_____
_____	_____

Cardio ☐   Strength ☐
Stretching ☐   Other ☐

Notes

_____
_____
_____

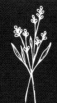 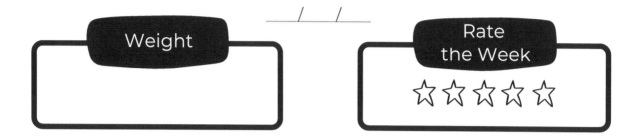 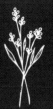

Week 9 Results

_____ / _____ / _____

Weight

Rate the Week
☆ ☆ ☆ ☆ ☆

What continues to be your hardest struggle at this point?
What changes do you still need to make to overcome this struggle?

_____
_____
_____
_____

What worked well this past week?

_____
_____
_____

What was challenging this past week?

_____
_____
_____

What is one thing you can improve this next week?

_____
_____
_____

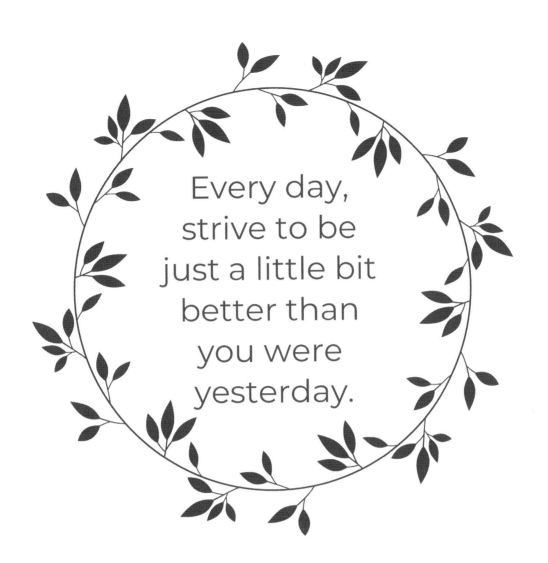

Every day,
strive to be
just a little bit
better than
you were
yesterday.

MY GOAL FOR THIS WEEK

_____

STEPS I WILL TAKE

_____

_____

_____

_____

Week Ten

	Breakfast	Lunch	Dinner	Snacks
Monday				
Tuesday				
Wednesday				
Thursday				
Friday				
Saturday				
Sunday				

Week Ten / Meal Plan

Sleep

7pm · 8 · 9 · 10 · 11 · 12am · 1 · 2 · 3 · 4 · 5 · 6 · 7 · 8 · 9 · 10 · 11 · 12pm

Quality: ☆☆☆☆☆   Hours: _____   Energy Level: ☆☆☆☆☆

Mood

| cheerful | sad | excited | worried | stressed |
| upset | angry | frustrated | content | indifferent |

Meals

BREAKFAST
_____
_____
_____

LUNCH
_____
_____
_____

DINNER
_____
_____
_____

SNACKS
_____
_____

Misc.

WATER: ▢ ▢ ▢ ▢ ▢ ▢ ▢ ▢

VITAMINS / SUPPLEMENTS ▢

STEPS: _____

OTHER: _____

Exercise

ACTIVITY	DISTANCE / REPS / TIME
_____	_____
_____	_____
_____	_____
_____	_____

Cardio ▢   Strength ▢
Stretching ▢   Other ▢

Notes

_____
_____
_____

Date _____ Tuesday

Sleep

7pm · 8 · 9 · 10 · 11 · 12am · 1 · 2 · 3 · 4 · 5 · 6 · 7 · 8 · 9 · 10 · 11 · 12pm

Quality: ☆ ☆ ☆ ☆ ☆   Hours: _____   Energy Level: ☆ ☆ ☆ ☆ ☆

Mood

| cheerful | sad | excited | worried | stressed |
| upset | angry | frustrated | content | indifferent |

Meals

BREAKFAST

LUNCH

DINNER

SNACKS

Misc.

WATER: ▯ ▯ ▯ ▯ ▯ ▯ ▯ ▯

VITAMINS / SUPPLEMENTS ☐

STEPS: _____

OTHER: _____

Exercise

ACTIVITY	DISTANCE / REPS / TIME

Cardio ☐   Strength ☐
Stretching ☐   Other ☐

Notes

Date

Wednesday

Sleep

7pm · 8 · 9 · 10 · 11 · 12am · 1 · 2 · 3 · 4 · 5 · 6 · 7 · 8 · 9 · 10 · 11 · 12pm

Quality: ☆☆☆☆☆   Hours: _____   Energy Level: ☆☆☆☆☆

Mood

| cheerful | sad | excited | worried | stressed |
| upset | angry | frustrated | content | indifferent |

Meals

BREAKFAST
_____
_____
_____
_____

LUNCH
_____
_____
_____
_____

DINNER
_____
_____
_____
_____

SNACKS
_____
_____
_____

Misc.

WATER: ☐ ☐ ☐ ☐ ☐ ☐ ☐ ☐

VITAMINS / SUPPLEMENTS ☐

STEPS: _____

OTHER: _____

Exercise

ACTIVITY	DISTANCE / REPS / TIME
_____	_____
_____	_____
_____	_____

Cardio ☐   Strength ☐
Stretching ☐   Other ☐

Notes

_____
_____
_____

Date

Thursday

_____

Sleep

7pm · 8 · 9 · 10 · 11 · 12am · 1 · 2 · 3 · 4 · 5 · 6 · 7 · 8 · 9 · 10 · 11 · 12pm

Quality: ☆☆☆☆☆   Hours: _____   Energy Level: ☆☆☆☆☆

Mood

| cheerful | sad | excited | worried | stressed |
| upset | angry | frustrated | content | indifferent |

Meals

BREAKFAST
_____
_____
_____

LUNCH
_____
_____
_____

DINNER
_____
_____
_____

SNACKS
_____
_____
_____

Misc.

WATER: ⬜ ⬜ ⬜ ⬜ ⬜ ⬜ ⬜ ⬜

VITAMINS / SUPPLEMENTS ☐

STEPS: _____

OTHER: _____

Exercise

ACTIVITY	DISTANCE / REPS / TIME
_____	_____
_____	_____
_____	_____
_____	_____

Cardio ☐   Strength ☐
Stretching ☐   Other ☐

Notes

_____
_____
_____

Sleep

7pm · 8 · 9 · 10 · 11 · 12am · 1 · 2 · 3 · 4 · 5 · 6 · 7 · 8 · 9 · 10 · 11 · 12pm

Quality: ☆☆☆☆☆   Hours: _____   Energy Level: ☆☆☆☆☆

Mood

| cheerful | sad | excited | worried | stressed |
| upset | angry | frustrated | content | indifferent |

Meals

BREAKFAST

LUNCH

DINNER

SNACKS

Misc.

WATER: ⬜⬜⬜⬜⬜⬜⬜⬜

VITAMINS / SUPPLEMENTS ☐

STEPS: _____

OTHER: _____

Exercise

ACTIVITY	DISTANCE / REPS / TIME

Cardio ☐   Strength ☐

Stretching ☐   Other ☐

Notes

Date

_____

Saturday

Sleep

7pm · 8 · 9 · 10 · 11 · 12am · 1 · 2 · 3 · 4 · 5 · 6 · 7 · 8 · 9 · 10 · 11 · 12pm

Quality: ☆☆☆☆☆   Hours: _____   Energy Level: ☆☆☆☆☆

Mood

| cheerful | sad | excited | worried | stressed |
| upset | angry | frustrated | content | indifferent |

Meals

BREAKFAST

LUNCH

DINNER

SNACKS

Misc.

WATER: ⊔ ⊔ ⊔ ⊔ ⊔ ⊔ ⊔ ⊔

VITAMINS / SUPPLEMENTS ☐

STEPS: _____

OTHER: _____

Exercise

ACTIVITY	DISTANCE / REPS / TIME

Cardio ☐   Strength ☐
Stretching ☐   Other ☐

Notes

Sleep

7pm · 8 · 9 · 10 · 11 · 12am · 1 · 2 · 3 · 4 · 5 · 6 · 7 · 8 · 9 · 10 · 11 · 12pm

Quality: ☆☆☆☆☆   Hours: _____   Energy Level: ☆☆☆☆☆

Mood

| cheerful | sad | excited | worried | stressed |
| upset | angry | frustrated | content | indifferent |

Meals

BREAKFAST

LUNCH

DINNER

SNACKS

Misc.

WATER: ▢▢▢▢▢▢▢▢

VITAMINS / SUPPLEMENTS ▢

STEPS: _____

OTHER: _____

Exercise

ACTIVITY	DISTANCE / REPS / TIME

Cardio ▢   Strength ▢

Stretching ▢   Other ▢

Notes

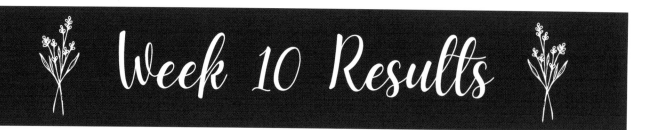

Week 10 Results

_____ / _____ / _____

Weight

Rate the Week

☆ ☆ ☆ ☆ ☆

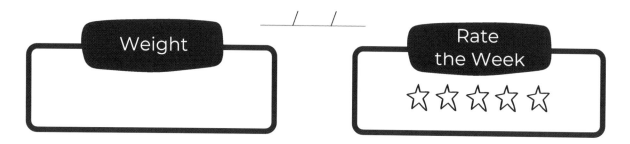

How can planning meals ahead of time help you avoid unhealthy choices?

_____

_____

_____

_____

What worked well this past week?

_____

_____

_____

What was challenging this past week?

_____

_____

_____

What is one thing you can improve this next week?

_____

_____

_____

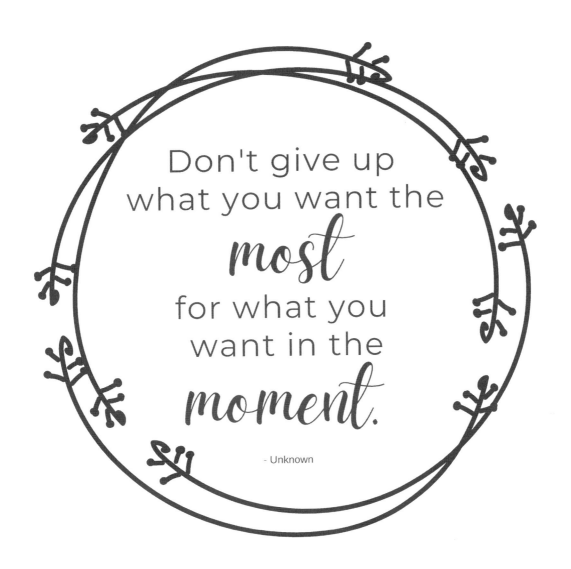

Don't give up
what you want the
most
for what you
want in the
moment.

- Unknown

MY GOAL FOR THIS WEEK

_____

STEPS I WILL TAKE

_____

_____

_____

Week Eleven

	Breakfast	Lunch	Dinner	Snacks
Monday				
Tuesday				
Wednesday				
Thursday				
Friday				
Saturday				
Sunday				

Week Eleven / Meal Plan

Date

Monday

Sleep

7pm · 8 · 9 · 10 · 11 · 12am · 1 · 2 · 3 · 4 · 5 · 6 · 7 · 8 · 9 · 10 · 11 · 12pm

Quality: ☆ ☆ ☆ ☆ ☆   Hours: _____   Energy Level: ☆ ☆ ☆ ☆ ☆

Mood

| cheerful | sad | excited | worried | stressed |
| upset | angry | frustrated | content | indifferent |

Meals

BREAKFAST

LUNCH

DINNER

SNACKS

Misc.

WATER: ⊔ ⊔ ⊔ ⊔ ⊔ ⊔ ⊔ ⊔

VITAMINS / SUPPLEMENTS ☐

STEPS: _____

OTHER: _____

Exercise

| ACTIVITY | DISTANCE / REPS / TIME |

Cardio ☐   Strength ☐

Stretching ☐   Other ☐

Notes

Date

Tuesday

Sleep

7pm · 8 · 9 · 10 · 11 · 12am · 1 · 2 · 3 · 4 · 5 · 6 · 7 · 8 · 9 · 10 · 11 · 12pm

Quality: ☆☆☆☆☆   Hours: _____   Energy Level: ☆☆☆☆☆

Mood

| cheerful | sad | excited | worried | stressed |
| upset | angry | frustrated | content | indifferent |

Meals

BREAKFAST

LUNCH

DINNER

SNACKS

Misc.

WATER: ⬜⬜⬜⬜⬜⬜⬜⬜

VITAMINS / SUPPLEMENTS ⬜

STEPS: _____

OTHER: _____

Exercise

ACTIVITY	DISTANCE / REPS / TIME

Cardio ⬜   Strength ⬜
Stretching ⬜   Other ⬜

Notes

Sleep

7pm · 8 · 9 · 10 · 11 · 12am · 1 · 2 · 3 · 4 · 5 · 6 · 7 · 8 · 9 · 10 · 11 · 12pm

Quality: ☆☆☆☆☆   Hours: _____   Energy Level: ☆☆☆☆☆

Mood

cheerful	sad	excited	worried	stressed
upset	angry	frustrated	content	indifferent

Meals

BREAKFAST

LUNCH

DINNER

SNACKS

Misc.

WATER: ▯ ▯ ▯ ▯ ▯ ▯ ▯ ▯

VITAMINS / SUPPLEMENTS ☐

STEPS: _____

OTHER: _____

Exercise

ACTIVITY	DISTANCE / REPS / TIME

Cardio ☐   Strength ☐

Stretching ☐   Other ☐

Notes

Date _____

Thursday

Sleep

7pm · 8 · 9 · 10 · 11 · 12am · 1 · 2 · 3 · 4 · 5 · 6 · 7 · 8 · 9 · 10 · 11 · 12pm

Quality: ☆☆☆☆☆   Hours: _____   Energy Level: ☆☆☆☆☆

Mood

| cheerful | sad | excited | worried | stressed |
| upset | angry | frustrated | content | indifferent |

Meals

BREAKFAST
_____
_____
_____
_____

LUNCH
_____
_____
_____
_____

DINNER
_____
_____
_____
_____

SNACKS
_____
_____

Misc.

WATER: ⬜⬜⬜⬜⬜⬜⬜⬜

VITAMINS / SUPPLEMENTS ☐

STEPS: _____

OTHER: _____

Exercise

ACTIVITY	DISTANCE / REPS / TIME
_____	_____
_____	_____
_____	_____
_____	_____

Cardio ☐   Strength ☐
Stretching ☐   Other ☐

Notes

_____
_____
_____

118 / Week Eleven

Date

_____

Friday

Sleep

7pm · 8 · 9 · 10 · 11 · 12am · 1 · 2 · 3 · 4 · 5 · 6 · 7 · 8 · 9 · 10 · 11 · 12pm

Quality: ☆☆☆☆☆   Hours: _____   Energy Level: ☆☆☆☆☆

Mood

cheerful   sad   excited   worried   stressed
upset   angry   frustrated   content   indifferent

Meals

BREAKFAST
_____
_____
_____
_____

LUNCH
_____
_____
_____
_____

DINNER
_____
_____
_____
_____

SNACKS
_____
_____
_____

Misc.

WATER: ▢ ▢ ▢ ▢ ▢ ▢ ▢ ▢

VITAMINS / SUPPLEMENTS ▢

STEPS: _____

OTHER: _____

Exercise

ACTIVITY	DISTANCE / REPS / TIME
_____	_____
_____	_____
_____	_____
_____	_____

Cardio ▢   Strength ▢
Stretching ▢   Other ▢

Notes

_____
_____
_____

Date

Sleep

7pm · 8 · 9 · 10 · 11 · 12am · 1 · 2 · 3 · 4 · 5 · 6 · 7 · 8 · 9 · 10 · 11 · 12pm

Quality: ☆☆☆☆☆   Hours: _____   Energy Level: ☆☆☆☆☆

Mood

| cheerful | sad | excited | worried | stressed |
| upset | angry | frustrated | content | indifferent |

Meals

BREAKFAST

LUNCH

DINNER

SNACKS

Misc.

WATER: ⬜⬜⬜⬜⬜⬜⬜⬜

VITAMINS / SUPPLEMENTS ☐

STEPS: _____

OTHER: _____

Exercise

ACTIVITY	DISTANCE / REPS / TIME

Cardio ☐   Strength ☐
Stretching ☐   Other ☐

Notes

Date _____

Sunday

Sleep

7pm · 8 · 9 · 10 · 11 · 12am · 1 · 2 · 3 · 4 · 5 · 6 · 7 · 8 · 9 · 10 · 11 · 12pm

Quality: ☆ ☆ ☆ ☆ ☆   Hours: _____   Energy Level: ☆ ☆ ☆ ☆ ☆

Mood

| cheerful | sad | excited | worried | stressed |
| upset | angry | frustrated | content | indifferent |

Meals

BREAKFAST

LUNCH

DINNER

SNACKS

Misc.

WATER: ⊔ ⊔ ⊔ ⊔ ⊔ ⊔ ⊔ ⊔

VITAMINS / SUPPLEMENTS ☐

STEPS: _____

OTHER: _____

Exercise

ACTIVITY	DISTANCE / REPS / TIME

Cardio ☐   Strength ☐
Stretching ☐   Other ☐

Notes

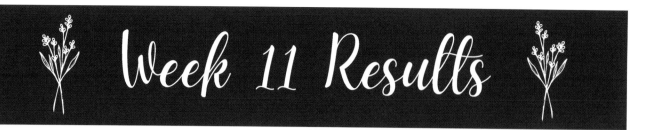

Week 11 Results

_____ / _____ / _____

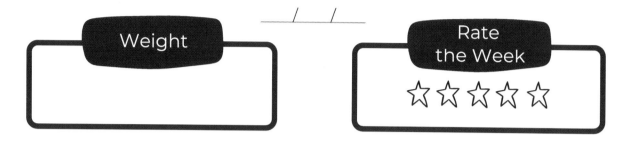

Weight

Rate
the Week

☆ ☆ ☆ ☆ ☆

What are 2-3 activities you would better enjoy with a healthier body?

_____

_____

_____

_____

What worked well this past week?

_____

_____

_____

What was challenging this past week?

_____

_____

_____

What is one thing you can improve this next week?

_____

_____

_____

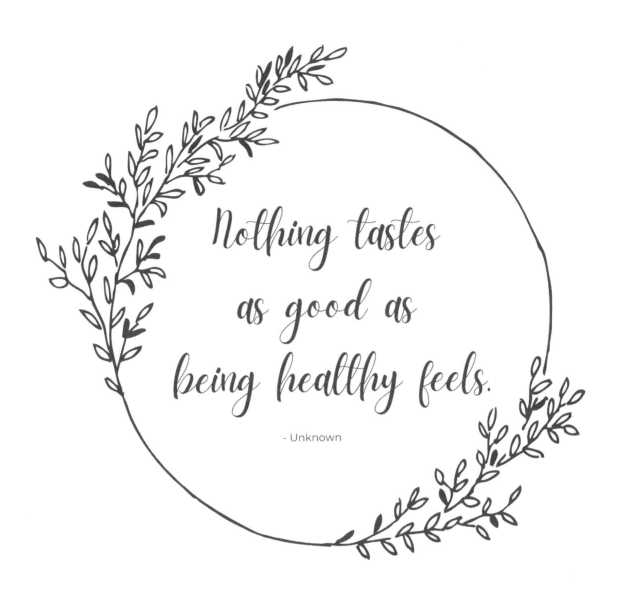

Nothing tastes as good as being healthy feels.

— Unknown

MY GOAL FOR THIS WEEK

_____

STEPS I WILL TAKE

_____

_____

_____

Week Twelve

	Breakfast	Lunch	Dinner	Snacks
Monday				
Tuesday				
Wednesday				
Thursday				
Friday				
Saturday				
Sunday				

Week Twelve / Meal Plan

Date ------- *Monday*

_____

Sleep

7pm · 8 · 9 · 10 · 11 · 12am · 1 · 2 · 3 · 4 · 5 · 6 · 7 · 8 · 9 · 10 · 11 · 12pm

Quality: ☆☆☆☆☆   Hours: _____   Energy Level: ☆☆☆☆☆

Mood

| cheerful | sad | excited | worried | stressed |
| upset | angry | frustrated | content | indifferent |

Meals

BREAKFAST
_____
_____
_____

LUNCH
_____
_____
_____

DINNER
_____
_____
_____

SNACKS
_____
_____
_____

Misc.

WATER: ⬜⬜⬜⬜⬜⬜⬜⬜

VITAMINS / SUPPLEMENTS ⬜

STEPS: _____

OTHER: _____

Exercise

ACTIVITY	DISTANCE / REPS / TIME
_____	_____
_____	_____
_____	_____

Cardio ⬜   Strength ⬜
Stretching ⬜   Other ⬜

Notes

_____
_____
_____

Date

tuesday

_____

Sleep

7pm · 8 · 9 · 10 · 11 · 12am · 1 · 2 · 3 · 4 · 5 · 6 · 7 · 8 · 9 · 10 · 11 · 12pm

Quality: ☆☆☆☆☆   Hours: _____   Energy Level: ☆☆☆☆☆

Mood

| cheerful | sad | excited | worried | stressed |
| upset | angry | frustrated | content | indifferent |

Meals

BREAKFAST

LUNCH

DINNER

SNACKS

Misc.

WATER: ▯ ▯ ▯ ▯ ▯ ▯ ▯ ▯

VITAMINS / SUPPLEMENTS ☐

STEPS: _____

OTHER: _____

Exercise

ACTIVITY	DISTANCE / REPS / TIME

Cardio ☐   Strength ☐

Stretching ☐   Other ☐

Notes

Wednesday

Sleep

7pm · 8 · 9 · 10 · 11 · 12am · 1 · 2 · 3 · 4 · 5 · 6 · 7 · 8 · 9 · 10 · 11 · 12pm

Quality: ☆ ☆ ☆ ☆ ☆   Hours: _____   Energy Level: ☆ ☆ ☆ ☆ ☆

Mood

| cheerful | sad | excited | worried | stressed |
| upset | angry | frustrated | content | indifferent |

Meals

BREAKFAST

LUNCH

DINNER

SNACKS

Misc.

WATER: ☐ ☐ ☐ ☐ ☐ ☐ ☐ ☐

VITAMINS / SUPPLEMENTS ☐

STEPS: _____

OTHER: _____

Exercise

ACTIVITY	DISTANCE / REPS / TIME

Cardio ☐   Strength ☐
Stretching ☐   Other ☐

Notes

Date _____

Sleep

7pm · 8 · 9 · 10 · 11 · 12am · 1 · 2 · 3 · 4 · 5 · 6 · 7 · 8 · 9 · 10 · 11 · 12pm

Quality: ☆☆☆☆☆   Hours: _____   Energy Level: ☆☆☆☆☆

Mood

| cheerful | sad | excited | worried | stressed |
| upset | angry | frustrated | content | indifferent |

Meals

BREAKFAST

LUNCH

DINNER

SNACKS

Misc.

WATER: ⬚ ⬚ ⬚ ⬚ ⬚ ⬚ ⬚ ⬚

VITAMINS / SUPPLEMENTS ☐

STEPS: _____

OTHER: _____

Exercise

ACTIVITY	DISTANCE / REPS / TIME

Cardio ☐   Strength ☐

Stretching ☐   Other ☐

Notes

Date _____ · · · Friday

Sleep

7pm · 8 · 9 · 10 · 11 · 12am · 1 · 2 · 3 · 4 · 5 · 6 · 7 · 8 · 9 · 10 · 11 · 12pm

Quality: ☆☆☆☆☆   Hours: _____   Energy Level: ☆☆☆☆☆

Mood

cheerful   sad   excited   worried   stressed
upset   angry   frustrated   content   indifferent

Meals

BREAKFAST

LUNCH

DINNER

SNACKS

Misc.

WATER: ☐☐☐☐☐☐☐☐

VITAMINS / SUPPLEMENTS ☐

STEPS: _____

OTHER: _____

Exercise

ACTIVITY	DISTANCE / REPS / TIME

Cardio ☐   Strength ☐
Stretching ☐   Other ☐

Notes

Date _____ Saturday

Sleep

7pm · 8 · 9 · 10 · 11 · 12am · 1 · 2 · 3 · 4 · 5 · 6 · 7 · 8 · 9 · 10 · 11 · 12pm

Quality: ☆☆☆☆☆   Hours: _____   Energy Level: ☆☆☆☆☆

Mood

| cheerful | sad | excited | worried | stressed |
| upset | angry | frustrated | content | indifferent |

Meals

BREAKFAST

LUNCH

DINNER

SNACKS

Misc.

WATER: ▯ ▯ ▯ ▯ ▯ ▯ ▯ ▯

VITAMINS / SUPPLEMENTS ☐

STEPS: _____

OTHER: _____

Exercise

ACTIVITY	DISTANCE / REPS / TIME

Cardio ☐   Strength ☐
Stretching ☐   Other ☐

Notes

Sunday

Sleep

7pm · 8 · 9 · 10 · 11 · 12am · 1 · 2 · 3 · 4 · 5 · 6 · 7 · 8 · 9 · 10 · 11 · 12pm

Quality: ☆☆☆☆☆   Hours: _____   Energy Level: ☆☆☆☆☆

Mood

| cheerful | sad | excited | worried | stressed |
| upset | angry | frustrated | content | indifferent |

Meals

BREAKFAST

LUNCH

DINNER

SNACKS

Misc.

WATER: ⬜⬜⬜⬜⬜⬜⬜⬜

VITAMINS / SUPPLEMENTS ☐

STEPS: _____

OTHER: _____

Exercise

ACTIVITY	DISTANCE / REPS / TIME

Cardio ☐   Strength ☐
Stretching ☐   Other ☐

Notes

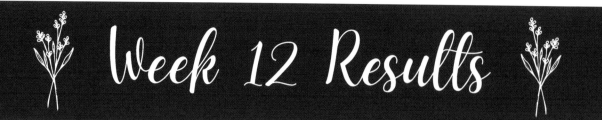

Week 12 Results

_____ / _____ / _____

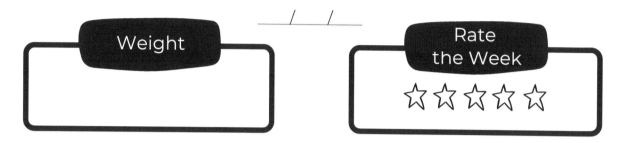

Weight		Rate the Week
		☆ ☆ ☆ ☆ ☆

Write a brief note to your old self, thanking her for making the choices that brought you to this point.

_____

_____

_____

_____

_____

_____

_____

How can your family and friends continue to support your new lifestyle? Please share your thoughts with them.

_____

_____

_____

Why is it important that you continue to focus on and make your new, healthier lifestyle a priority?

_____

_____

_____

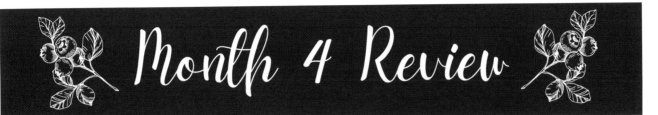

Month 4 Review

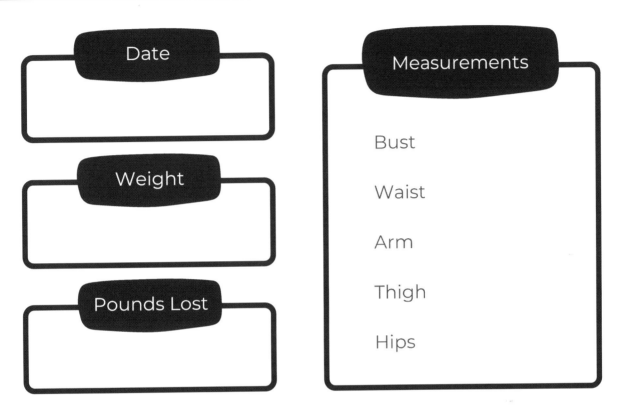

Date

Weight

Pounds Lost

Measurements

Bust

Waist

Arm

Thigh

Hips

List a success or accomplishment you're proud of from this month.

_____

List any old habits that are still a struggle.

_____

_____

_____

What habits do you need to focus on and prioritize moving forward?

_____

_____

_____

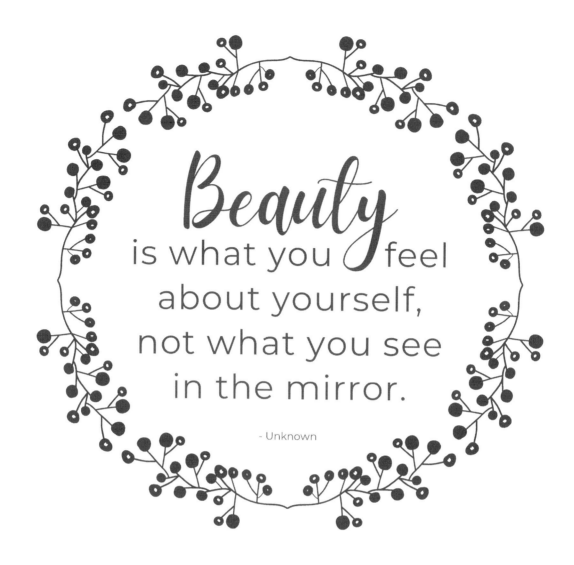

Beauty is what you feel about yourself, not what you see in the mirror.

- Unknown

What are you most proud of from this journey?

_____

_____

_____

_____

What changes have you noticed in your body and your physical health?

_____

_____

_____

_____

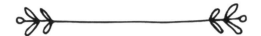

BEFORE & AFTER PAGE

MEASUREMENT TRACKERS

WEEKLY WEIGH-IN TRACKER

POUNDS LOST TRACKER

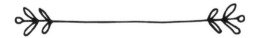

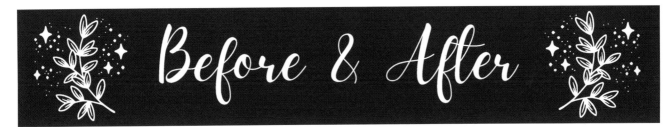

Before & After

Date

Date

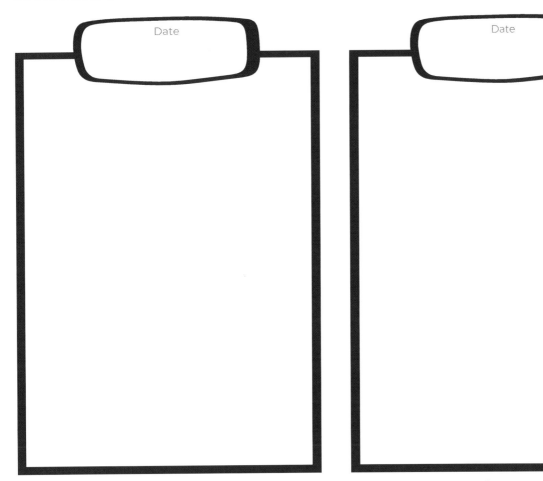

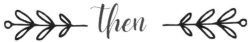 Then

Now

Then	Now
Weight	Weight
Bust	Bust
Waist	Waist
Arm	Arm
Thigh	Thigh
Hips	Hips

Total pounds lost: _____

Total inches lost: _____

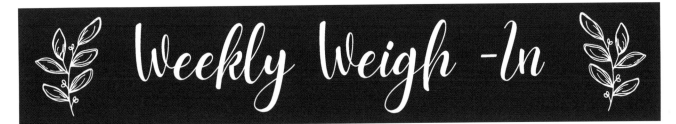

Weekly Weigh -In

Week 1

_____
Weight

+ / - _____ lbs

_____
Total lbs lost

Week 2

_____
Weight

+ / - _____ lbs

_____
Total lbs lost

Week 3

_____
Weight

+ / - _____ lbs

_____
Total lbs lost

Week 4

_____
Weight

+ / - _____ lbs

_____
Total lbs lost

Week 5

_____
Weight

+ / - _____ lbs

_____
Total lbs lost

Week 6

_____
Weight

+ / - _____ lbs

_____
Total lbs lost

Week 7

_____
Weight

+ / - _____ lbs

_____
Total lbs lost

Week 8

_____
Weight

+ / - _____ lbs

_____
Total lbs lost

Week 9

_____
Weight

+ / - _____ lbs

_____
Total lbs lost

Week 10

_____
Weight

+ / - _____ lbs

_____
Total lbs lost

Week 11

_____
Weight

+ / - _____ lbs

_____
Total lbs lost

Week 12

_____
Weight

+ / - _____ lbs

_____
Total lbs lost

Even slow progress gets you a step closer to success!

Pounds Lost

1	2	3	4	5	6	7	8	9	10
11	12	13	14	15	16	17	18	19	20
21	22	23	24	25	26	27	28	29	30
31	32	33	34	35	36	37	38	39	40
41	42	43	44	45	46	47	48	49	50
51	52	53	54	55	56	57	58	59	60
61	62	63	64	65	66	67	68	69	70
71	72	73	74	75	76	77	78	79	80
81	82	83	84	85	86	87	88	89	90
91	92	93	94	95	96	97	98	99	100

A little progress each day adds up to big results!
- Unknown

Measurement tracker

Week 1
Bust
Waist
Arm
Thigh
Hips

Week 2
Bust
Waist
Arm
Thigh
Hips

Week 3
Bust
Waist
Arm
Thigh
Hips

Week 4
Bust
Waist
Arm
Thigh
Hips

Week 5
Bust
Waist
Arm
Thigh
Hips

Week 6
Bust
Waist
Arm
Thigh
Hips

Week 7
Bust
Waist
Arm
Thigh
Hips

Week 8
Bust
Waist
Arm
Thigh
Hips

Week 9
Bust
Waist
Arm
Thigh
Hips

Week 10
Bust
Waist
Arm
Thigh
Hips

Week 11
Bust
Waist
Arm
Thigh
Hips

Week 12
Bust
Waist
Arm
Thigh
Hips

Measurement tracker

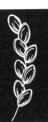

Month 1
Bust
Waist
Arm
Thigh
Hips

Month 2
Bust
Waist
Arm
Thigh
Hips

Month 3
Bust
Waist
Arm
Thigh
Hips

Month 4
Bust
Waist
Arm
Thigh
Hips

Month 5
Bust
Waist
Arm
Thigh
Hips

Month 6
Bust
Waist
Arm
Thigh
Hips

Month 7
Bust
Waist
Arm
Thigh
Hips

Month 8
Bust
Waist
Arm
Thigh
Hips

Month 9
Bust
Waist
Arm
Thigh
Hips

Month 10
Bust
Waist
Arm
Thigh
Hips

Month 11
Bust
Waist
Arm
Thigh
Hips

Month 12
Bust
Waist
Arm
Thigh
Hips

You don't have to be extreme, just consistent.
- Unknown

Made in the USA
Columbia, SC
13 October 2024

44221107R00085